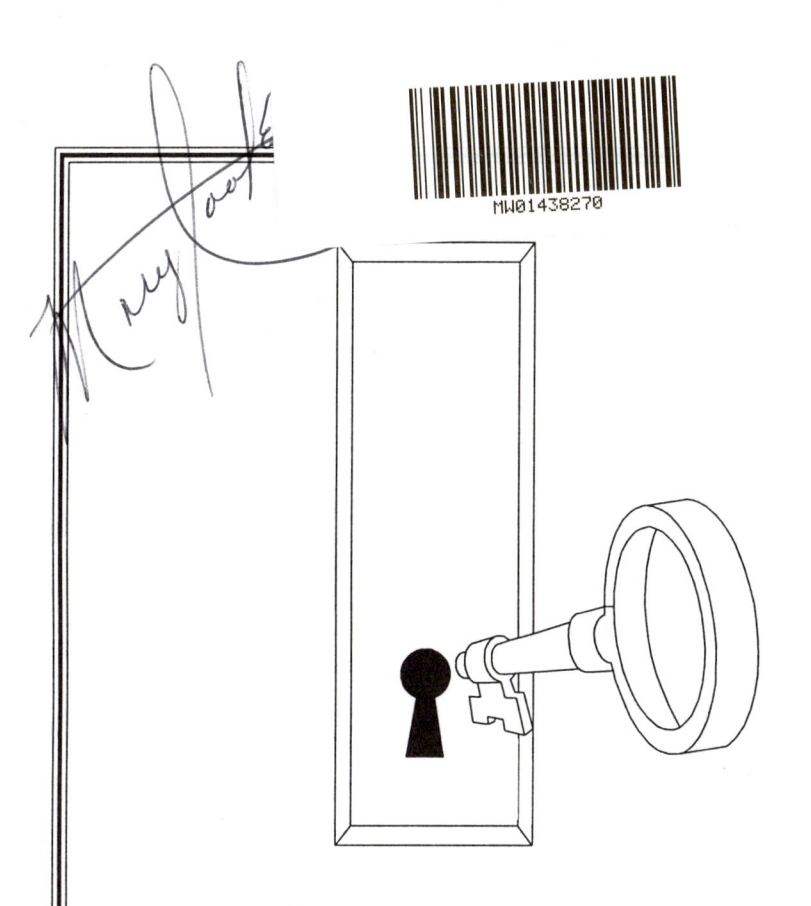

I Carried A Key

Three Years In A Mental Hospital:
A Nurse's Story

by Agnes MacKinnon

I Carried A Key
Three Years in a Mental Hospital: A Nurse's Story

Copyright © 1996 Agnes Eva MacKinnon

All rights reserved. No portion of this book may be duplicated in any way without the expressed written consent of the author.

ISBN: 0-9680498-0-X

First Printing

Desktop publishing production and editing by Ken Morisette.
Printed in Canada by Hignell Printing Limited.
Distributed by Sandhill Book Marketing.

This book is historical fiction based on the author's experience of nursing training in the British Columbia Provincial Mental Hospital at Essondale, now known as Riverview Hospital. With the exception of some admirable medical and senior nursing staff, all names and characters in the book are fictional. Where names of real people are used, it is in recognition of their dedication and good work.

Acknowledgements

All incidents related in this book were actual happenings. With a few notable exceptions, fictional names are used for the nursing staff; the Administrative and Medical staff are those of the early `30s.

The author is deeply grateful to members of the Riverview Historical Committee and to John I. Yarske, former Chief Executive Officer of Riverview Hospital; to Dr. Barry Ledwidge who brought the manuscript to the attention of these members; to David Davies, instructor, who provided access to the pictures taken by the official hospital photographer; to Anna Tremere, Head Nurse, and to Donna Higenbottam, Manager of Education Services, who were my contacts with the Historical Committee; to Ken Morisette, Information Officer, who assisted in preparing the manuscript; as did Laurie Hilborn, typist. Brian Young, Provincial Archivist in Victoria, provided statistics. I particularly thank my granddaughter, Stephanie Roberts, who was the catalyst in bringing my manuscript to the attention of Historical Committee members at Riverview Hospital.

Dedication

Dedicated to the memory of my husband, Neil MacKinnon, who gave me constant loving support.

KEYS

They click, click, click all the day,
They click, click, click all the night.
I don't understand what it means!
They keep me awake with fright.
Some open doors and windows,
Some open cupboards and racks;
But the best way to escape from this building
Is to slide if you can through the cracks.
Keys to the right of us, keys to the left of us,
Keys at both ends of the hall;
But the door has not yet been found
That needs no key at all.
A bobbed haired maiden has charge of those keys,
They are strung round her waist on a belt,
And if you say no when she says yes
Her displeasure may surely be felt.
It's all very well to brag and boast
Of a grand new hospital so near the coast,
But a broken heart it will not mend
Nor a lost soul to heaven send.
And more's the pity in any case
For God never intended there be such a place.

Written by a patient in the Provincial Mental Hospital at Essondale
circa 1934.

CHAPTER ONE

The last heavy metal door clanged shut behind me. I was locked into a ward of deranged women in the Provincial Mental Hospital at Essondale, which most people called the Insane Asylum. I was only 16 years old, and my first day as a psychiatric nurse had begun.

A confused impression of restlessness and the hubbub of nearly one hundred disturbed souls struck instant terror into my heart, and I instinctively backed up against the wall of the dayroom as protection from the surreptitious attack that seemed inevitable. What bizarre circumstances had led to this threatening situation?

The other nurses had scattered to their accustomed duties, but I could not make my feet in their squeaky new white shoes move to follow them. In my panic I wondered how I would ever survive the 12-hour day that stretched before me. My hand crept through the opening on the side of the crisp white nurse's apron that symbolized my supposed authority over the unfortunate women in this institution, and I closed my fingers around the heavy key that rested in my uniform pocket. That key represented freedom; it would open the doors that led to the outside. The thought comforted me and I relaxed enough to timidly survey the strange surroundings.

Amazingly, the inmates paid little attention to the newest probationer flattened against the dayroom wall. Some of the women huddled in chairs or settees around the large room; others were constantly on the move as their inner demons drove them to frantic mutterings or wailing cries of wretchedness and dispair. These minds were trapped by the false but unshakable delusions that led to their imprisonment within asylum walls.

Barely an hour had passed since the steady ringing of a hand bell at the bottom of the stairs in the Nurses' Home awakened the occupants of the eight-bed dormitory where I had spent a restless night in a strange bed, my mind a turmoil of uncertainty and doubt. As the girls I had met for the first time last night stirred and began their morning routines, I struggled out of my twisted sheets and straightened the bed while watching for a chance to wash up at one of the two basins in a corner of the room.

The moment came to sort out the various pieces of heavily-starched cotton that were a feature of pre-nylon uniforms in my youth. Obviously the blue uniform dress went on first.

"D'you have enough safety pins?" Fully dressed with the ease of two weeks of practice, the sturdily-built girl who had taken me under her wing last night after my inauspicious introduction to the dormitory by the fussy Night Supervisor, came to my assistance. Her brown hair was cut short in a boyish bob, softened by a spit curl on each side of her forehead, her only concession to feminine vanity. Her freckled face was free of make-up and shone with good will. I turned to Gladwin gratefully, as she picked up the square probationer's bib and a couple of pins.

"Always pin the bib through the waistband of your dress to anchor it down," she instructed, suiting her actions to her words. She turned me around. "Cross the straps at the back before you pin them down. Now the key-belt. No, don't put it around your waist. Wear it lower, over your hips, and have the strap with the key on it on the right side so you can drop the key into the pocket of your dress." The thick leather belt rested heavily on my hips and the responsibility it represented weighed on my spirits. There was little time for anxiety though as the girls around me finished their toilettes, transformed from the carefree girls of last night to white-clad guardians of unpredictable unstable personalities. Their matter-of-fact bearing and cheerful countenances lessened the fears that had plagued me since I had been swept into this menacing environment.

Gladwin was pinning the overlapping ends of the all-enveloping starched apron at the back. "Be sure the pins go through the waistband," she said. "You don't want the apron slipping around so the slit to reach your pocket isn't lined up properly. Now for the belt that covers all these safety pins. Did you bring studs to fasten it?"

My dresser mirror reflected an image of instant professionalism and the glow of satisfaction provided by this knowledge accompanied me as I followed Gladwin down the stairs to the large living room on the main floor where the nurses were gathering for roll call.

Though we were not the first to arrive there were still easy chairs to sink into while we waited. I observed the scene with interest.

Not everyone sat quietly around us. Some of the girls went through to the kitchen for a quick cup of coffee, for we went on duty without breakfast. Others made a bee-line for the door at the end of the room, which Gladwin told me led to the smoking room. "No smoking in the bedrooms," she told me. "You don't smoke, do you? Neither do I."

At some signal I didn't catch, lines began forming facing the entrance from the center hall of the Nurses' Home. The immaculately-clad Superintendent of Nurses and her assistant, Miss Marlatt, entered and stood at the front of the room. I recognized Miss Hicks, dark-haired and bright-eyed, as she had interviewed me less than a week ago and phoned the next day to tell me I was hired.

Gladwin had taken her place at the end of a line with a murmured, "Just wait until your name is called. We line up in order of seniority." I felt very conspicuous standing awkwardly to one side as the roll call proceeded.

Miss Marlatt, in striking contrast to Miss Hicks, was very fair, with fine blond hair softly waved ending in a neat roll below her ears. She was calling the names of each ward staff in turn from a ledger, marking them present as they responded, "Here." As soon as a ward list was complete, the Charge Nurse at the head of the line led her staff out the front door for the walk over to the main buildings. I noticed that Miss Hicks inspected each girl thoroughly as she passed by on her way out. She would allow no stocking runs or crooked seams, no unevenly pinned hems, no sign of anything less than the professional exactitude which she herself personified. She had set up this training school for psychiatric nurses and her standards were high.

Most of the nurses had left and my name had not yet been called. Gladwin's line was one of the two still present and I began to hope I would be with her on her ward. "Ward H2. Miss Coghlan, Miss

Richmond, Miss Dawson, Miss Gladwin, Miss Lehman!" I joined my friend thankfully and received Miss Hick's smile of encouragement as we passed her on the way to my first day on the wards. There was no backing out now. A feeling of inevitability had taken over, and I had my new friend Gladwin beside me. I was becoming accustomed to calling her by her last name, and being called Lehman in return....so that we won't make a mistake on the wards and call someone by her first name in front of patients, I had been told. They'd pick it up and we'd lose authority if they could use our first names.

Even at the early hour of a quarter to seven, on this spring morning the sun was warming the air as our procession made its way along the sidewalk past white two-storied square houses. The first white-clad groups were already halfway up the hillside approaching the ominous buildings that contained unknown dangers which lurked at the back of my mind. Gladwin chatted unconcernedly.

"These are doctors' and administrative staff houses," she informed me. "But not the most senior doctors. They're up on the hillside well above the institutional buildings, off by themselves." She gave a little giggle. "There's a real cute young doctor living in this house," and she pointed out a place we were passing. "Tall, and shy, and not married. But he's engaged." She sighed deeply and we both laughed.

As we started up the slope I asked Gladwin about the ward we would be on, which we would soon be entering. "H2 is a good ward," she assured me. "It's on the main floor. Probies are started on F2 or H2, the quietest wards. Wards F2, F3, and F4 are to the left of the main entrance; H2, H3, and H4 to the right. The higher you go the more disturbed the patients are, I'm told. They're not too bad on H2." We had climbed the front steps and were passing the offices that lined the entrance hall. The elevator doors at the end of the hall closed on a full load and the nurses left behind turned to the staircases on either side to go up to their wards.

I followed the H2 staff to the right and Miss Coghlan unlocked a door straight ahead of us. A shiver passed through me as the first door clanged shut behind me. "Welcome to ward H2," Gladwin smiled mischievously but with a sympathetic glance.

We were in a long empty corridor lined with locked doors on

either side, leading to a square room furnished with a table and comfortable chairs set on a wool rug. It looked like an ordinary sitting room, and it, too, was empty. "The rotunda," Gladwin told me. "It's at the center of the ward. The dormitories are through that door," pointing to the left, "and the dayrooms on the right. There's another staircase through those doors straight ahead. We go into the office first for the night report." She turned sharp right and we followed the three senior nurses into a small room with a window overlooking the courtyard between our ward and the main offices. What drew my eyes, though, was a large window on another wall that made it possible to supervise the dayroom from this room. Only the glass separated us from the women to be seen on the other side.

Two sleepy nurses finishing a 12-hour night shift had stood up as Miss Coghlan entered and seated herself behind the desk. Brisk and authoritative, she wore the same wide bib as senior nurses Dawson and Richmond, but the sleeves of her blue uniform were long and edged with starched cuffs. Her cap was edged with two black bands, marking her as a full-fledged psychiatric nurse, hence her position as Charge of a ward. The rest of the staff, including night nurses, stood in her presence. I placed myself along a wall beside Gladwin.

Stewart, the senior night nurse, read her report aloud. They had a routine night except for one item. "Mrs. Ridley was restless and agitated...."

Miss Coghlan interrupted. "Couldn't you have ordered a tranquilizer when the doctor made his rounds?"

"She didn't become disturbed until after Dr. Jackson was here," explained Stewart. She continued reading her report. "Mrs. Ridley is dressed this morning, sitting in the dayroom though she is very disturbed." She finished her report and there were no further comments.

Before going into the dayroom with Stewart to make the count, for the night staff could not go off duty until the whereabouts of every patient was known, Miss Coghlan assigned our duties.

"Richmond and Dawson, check the dormitories. Gladwin, the dayrooms. Lehman, stay with Gladwin to learn the routine." She preceded us into the first dayroom, and started slowly circling the room with Stewart.

"Never go ahead of a senior nurse," Gladwin explained as she followed the two Charge nurses. "And that means me, too. Even one day gives you seniority over anyone starting after you. It's silly, really, but boy! they take it seriously around here."

The office door clanged shut behind me with a reverberation that sent a shiver of panic right through me. I froze. Gladwin had disappeared through a door where I could see a room similar to this one, and the two nurses had progressed to the far end of the first dayroom with their count. Alone and afraid, I backed against a wall and felt for the key in my pocket.

As I realized that no one approached me my panic subsided somewhat, but the scene was confusing and the noise of many voices merged into a senseless babble. The count was now being made in the second dayroom and I wondered how it was managed with all the women moving about. Gladwin had not reappeared and a crowd was gathering at the door leading to the rotunda, not far from where I doggedly held my place.

My nerves jumped as a middle-aged woman spoke to me.

"You're new here, aren't you?" she said in a rush. "I can tell. There's been new nurses coming for summer relief. I know hospital routine; I worked in the Vancouver General."

Why, she's normal! I thought in relief. She looks normal and she sounds normal. I wonder what she's doing here?

But her voice was rising and her face becoming flushed as she continued to speak. "I don't belong here, you know. I'm not crazy. I was put here by the Devil and I wish he would leave me alone!" She began to wail, "He taunted and tormented me all night! Oh-Oh!" Her hands twisted and her body began to writhe in despair.

"Now, Mrs. Ridley, come along with me and I'll give you your medication before breakfast." Miss Coghlan was returning to the office with Stewart. "There's the buzzer now. Lehman, help Gladwin clear out the dayrooms, and check the washroom to see that nobody stays in there." A spacious washroom was located by the door of the second dayroom, where Gladwin appeared leading two apathetic women who did not seem to be interested in going for breakfast. I noticed that the toilet stalls had no doors.

The women congregated at the door were filing out, with Dawson at the rotunda door making a count as they passed her. "Richmond is counting at the dining room door," Gladwin told me as we herded the last of the women out of the dayrooms and followed them down the entrance corridor toward the main offices. I could see the women turning right at the end of the hall; the patients' dining room and the kitchens were directly behind the elevator and the main entrance. I asked Gladwin about the doors on either side of the hall that I had noticed when coming into the ward.

Gladwin named them as we passed. Utility room, clothes room, linens, kitchen - a small one for the ward, dispensary, visitors' room. I could now see Richmond making a count at the dining room door.

"Why all the counting?" I asked Gladwin. "They've been counted three times since we came on duty!"

"Oh, we have some slippery customers," Gladwin laughed. "If they don't feel like eating they'll slip back to the dormitories, or hide in a washroom. There aren't enough of us to keep an eye on every person all the time." We were now in the dining room and the corridor door banged shut behind us.

The women each picked up a divided metal plate and lined up at a gleaming stainless steel counter to receive her portion of cereal and toast, which she took to one of the long tables. Gladwin and I took coffee jugs and she led me to the ward H2 tables.

"There's four wards that eat here," she said. "H2 women are at the first four tables, and the next four are ward H3. Wards F2 and F3 are at the eight tables on the other side." I could see a dwindling lineup at a serving-counter opposite; most of the approximately four hundred women were already seated. Some had finished eating and were stealing food from the persons near them, who sometimes protested vigorously and sometimes didn't seem to care. The noise was now a confused roar.

Dawson came up to me as I was trying to fill coffee cups while dodging flailing arms and thrown pieces of food. Nurses were patrolling at every table, stopping to help uninterested eaters or to intervene in squabbles over food.

"Lehman, bring a plate of toast and see that Mrs. Ridley gets some. She's drowsy with medication and hasn't noticed that hers was taken." Snatches of sentences came to me as I went for the toast.

There were no conversations; mealtimes appeared to be a blend of quarrels over food, self-absorbed mumblings, and fanatical harangues directed to the world at large and nobody in particular.

"Nurse, Mrs. Smith is hogging all the toast again." I stopped to apportion the large woman's plateful of toast amongst her neighbors.

A stout woman sat regally at the head of the first table, looking disdainfully around her. Seeing my eyes upon her, she announced, "I'm Queen Victoria, and don't you forget it!" as she lifted her coffee cup with her little finger raised delicately in the air. Indeed she looked the part, wearing a full-skirted black dress that touched the floor, with her hair arranged on top of her head in the style of the last century. A musty smell surrounded her.

Mrs. Ridley was seated at a table but was not eating. I stopped to coax her with a piece of toast but she wailed, "Leave me alone! Oh, stop pestering me." She put her hands over her ears and rocked from side to side.

"She's listening to voices in her head," Richmond explained as she drew me away. "You can go to breakfast now, Lehman. Gladwin will show you where to go; she's waiting for you."

"We're lucky to get early breakfast," Gladwin said as she led me around a corner to the junior staff dining room, leaving the tumultuous noise and confusion out of sight but not out of sound. I realized I was hungry; it seemed like hours since we got out of bed.

"How long do we get for meals?" I inquired, taking in the fact that the half dozen girls at each table were eating quickly and hardly took time to glance at us.

"Half an hour for breakfast and the same for supper," said Gladwin, sliding into a chair and flapping a hand at the seat beside her. "And 45 minutes for dinner, at noon. You met Kelsey, Dunbar, and Langley last night in the dorm." The girls nodded and smiled.

A neat, gray-haired woman was at our side. "Do you want your eggs hard or soft?" she asked, setting a plate of toast in front of us. We stated our preference; she poured coffee for us and went out. Langley snorted.

"Hard or soft! What a laugh! They all come out of one pot; I've been out there when she picked them out." Her straight dark hair swung as she tossed her head in scorn. "Mrs. May is a dear, though. You'd never know she was a patient, would you?"

Fraser flopped into the last chair at our table. "Boy, am I late! I'm always late getting off F4. We hardly have time to eat, anyway. I'll have mine soft, thank you," to Mrs. May. We all laughed, and Fraser looked insulted.

"What's so funny? Cripes, am I sick of this place! Why did I have to get stuck on ward F4?" She scowled and wrinkled her nose, her mouth pulled down in discontent. Her hair was cut in bangs that reached her eyebrows, and she kept her eyelids down as if she could shut out the cruel world by not looking.

"What's ward F4 like?" Gladwin asked apprehensively. "I'm going to be moved any day now that Lehman's here." She looked at me and added quickly, "We all start on a lower floor to learn the ropes. Wards F4 and H4 are top floor, the worst of all except ward J, and it's all cells. Tell us about F4, Fraser."

"F4 is dirty! Oh, it's as clean as scrubbing can make it; Miss Keith sees to that! But the patients are dirty. They don't look after themselves; they have to be herded through the washroom after every meal. What a job! They don't even shower themselves, most of them. So that's divided up and there's showers every day at bedtime, and you have to almost get under the shower yourself. And some of them have open sores..."

"Spare us, Fraser. We'll be losing our breakfast," Dunbar spoke, wrinkling her nose in distaste.

"It's all right for you, Dunbar. You're on H4."

"Oh, yeah? That's the violent ward, I'll have you know. Let's get some fresh air; we still have a few minutes."

Heedlessly I started out, and Gladwin touched my arm. "Wait, Lehman. Seniority, remember?" I stepped aside and followed the others out to the front porch, where we found nurses sitting on the benches or the steps in the sunshine. Miss Coghlan was there, too, as well as other senior nurses. In just a few minutes a buzzer summoned us back to the wards and the doors clanged shut behind us again.

Miss Coghlan unlocked the dispensary door while giving us our duties. "Dormitories, Gladwin. Lehman, you'll be in the dayroom with Richmond, after she's had breakfast. Gladwin will stay with you until she comes back." She entered a spotless white room with medicine cupboards on one wall, and I saw a stretcher and other hospital equipment, before Gladwin and I went on to the dayrooms.

The women were quieter after their meal and Gladwin and I took turns escorting those who received medication down the hall to Miss Coghlan. "What are those different groups gathering at the rotunda door waiting for?" I asked Gladwin.

"Oh, they're the workers for the dormitories or dayroom cleaning," Gladwin explained. "I'll take my dormitory workers to the utility room to get brooms and mops, and pick up any linens we might need for the beds, when Richmond comes back. Dawson will take the O.T. ladies - you were up there when you were measured for uniforms, weren't you?"

"O.T.? That's Occupational Therapy, up in the attic, right? There's really a lot for the women to do, isn't there?"

"Some of ours are in the kitchen, too," Gladwin told me. "Mrs. May is one. She'll come back here soon, then someone takes her back for dinner and again for supper. She likes waiting on our tables. You know," Gladwin looked serious, "the ones who keep busy at something are better off than those who stay in the dayrooms, doing nothing but moan about their troubles." The clanging dayroom doors broadcast the return of the senior nurses, and Gladwin went to the rotunda door where she called, "Dormitory!" Nearly a dozen women followed her out.

Dawson called, "O.T.!" and took out another group, followed by Richmond, who said, "Dayroom! Come with us, Lehman. You'll be doing this by yourself in a few days."

At the utility room the women picked out cleaning supplies - mops, brooms, buckets of soapy water, paste wax, polishing cloths. And carpet sweepers. "No vacuum cleaners?" I asked. "Everything else is so up-to-date here you'd think there'd be vacuum cleaners."

"Too dangerous," was the succinct reply. "And speaking of up-to-date, look at our floor polishers!" Richmond smiled broadly.

Three or four women had picked out heavy flat blocks wrapped in old blanket cloth, and were pushing them up and down by their long handles on the hardwood floors.

"That monotonous activity suits some women and it goes on in the men's wards, too, I hear. You'll see those polishing blocks on every ward, at all hours, every day. I suppose it's kind of soothing; there must be something to it." We were back in the dayroom, with the cleaners going about their accustomed tasks. As we walked about I marvelled at the highly-polished floors and the gleaming furniture now being polished anew. Broadloom carpets, obviously especially made, covered most of the floor in each dayroom. Upholstered easy chairs and wooden settees lined the walls. On two sides were large windows barred into small panes and topped with scalloped valances. Framed pictures occupied all available wall spaces around the room.

Now that half the patients had left the dayrooms my initial panic subsided and a feeling of wonder at the attempts to alleviate an institutional atmosphere took its place in my mind.

"This must have cost a mint," I said to Richmond. "And it all looks so new."

"This building was opened about four years ago," Richmond told me. "It was finished just before the stock-market crash and patients were transferred from Number Nine in New Westminster and from the Acute Building. The government wasn't so lucky with the Veterans' Building, down by the main road. It's all finished, but stands empty. Not enough money to furnish it or pay staff." She mused for a minute. "I read somewhere that furnishings for this building alone cost $114,000. That's a lot of money." And so it was, in the 1930's.

Richmond was tall with a commanding upright presence. She had clear green eyes and a slight dusting of freckles across her nose. Her calmness and readiness to explain eased the terror I had felt upon first entering the ward; having to move amongst the women and finding myself unmolested quieted my fears though I still had misgivings about being left alone in this unpredictable setting. I stayed close to Richmond as she went into the washroom to check the cleaning in there. The busy women paid no attention to us.

"You probably wonder at the inmates doing the ward work," Richmond said, choosing a comfortable chair that commanded a view of both dayrooms. I drew one up beside her. "I was surprised too at first, but when you think about it, the women are much better off occupying themselves with familiar tasks rather than sitting around wringing their hands or turning into passive lumps, like some you see here. Some of these women have been institutionalized so long they've lost all initiative. They were moved here from Number Nine. You know - it's called Woodlands School now and houses just the retarded. They used to be out here, even the children, in with this type of patient. I'm sure Miss Hicks told you not to say 'the insane.' This is a mental hospital and houses mental patients."

A noisy woman on the porch off the dayroom drew us outside. Richmond continued her instruction as we walked out to her. "If these women were at home they'd be making beds and cleaning house. Even pushing a floor polisher gives them much needed exercise."

Richmond persuaded the noisy woman to climb down from the porch window bars and directed her to go out to the porch off the second dayroom, which faced away from the front entrance. "But no climbing on the bars," she reminded her firmly. "You know that's not allowed." The woman wandered off, muttering indistinctly to herself.

We were walking past 'Queen Victoria' who was seated majestically in a leather arm chair by the door to the porch. Her voluminous floor-length black skirts spread regally around her; the drawstrings of a capacious black cloth bag hung over her arm. She gave us a belligerent stare.

"Probably expects us to curtsy," I murmured.

Now out of her hearing, Richmond turned to me and said sharply, "Never ridicule or argue with a patient over her delusions. If she thinks she's Queen Victoria, nothing you say will persuade her differently. We call her 'Queenie' and she's quite satisfied with that, which is a little out of character when you think about it. But she's right on when it comes to taking a bath. She puts up an unholy row, so we mostly leave her alone. It's a major undertaking; we don't try it very often. Baths weren't popular in Queen Victoria's day, were they?"

I wouldn't like to have to persuade Queenie to do anything she didn't want to do, I agreed. She's a big woman.

"We'd all get into the act," Richmond pulled a wry face. "Don't forget, you're in charge here. If you don't keep control, you won't last. Never argue with an obsession. Don't threaten, and don't plead. We don't have to deal with unexpected violence on this ward; you'll learn how to control an unruly patient when you move to the upper floors. There are holds you can use that don't hurt them, and there are more nurses on the upper floors. Remember, we're not here to argue the patients out of their beliefs, no matter how silly they may seem. Don't provoke them to violence. O.K.?" I agreed hastily.

"What is Dawson doing this morning?" I asked. "I see her coming and going with several different patients." Short, bubbly Dawson was a marked contrast to Richmond in looks and in the way she moved. She bounced with pent-up energy where Richmond's bearing was impressively deliberate. Yet Dawson was undoubtedly in charge in her handling of the patients.

"Dawson is running errands," Richmond explained. "Picking up medications; the hospital dispensary is in the basement of the next building. Taking women over to pick up the ward laundry, and bringing folded and ironed linens down from the O.T. She'll bring the O.T. workers back for dinner, by the way. Then there are the appointments at the Beauty Parlor upstairs - did you notice it when you were taken up to be measured for uniforms? There's a dentist for the hospital, and a chiropodist. There might be a medical or psychiatric assessment, or hydrotherapy, or ultra violet lamp treatments. You'll go with one of us and learn your way around before you're assigned to another ward. I like doing errands; there's something different every day."

"You know, you sound like a teacher," I ventured.

"Actually, I took Normal School before I came here, but I haven't been lucky enough to get a school yet. I didn't apply out of the Lower Mainland area the first year; some of my friends are teaching in outlying districts and it looks like I'll have to start there too. Meanwhile the pay here is about the same when you figure room and board, and we get far more than nurses in training schools in general hospitals. We get the same subjects as they do in our lectures, with psychiatry as well."

"Surely teaching pays better than this," I exclaimed. "Doesn't it?"

"Not really," Richmond said. "I have a cousin who teaches in

Saskatchewan, and she's working for room and board, just to get experience. The parents board the teacher in turn, so she has to move every few months and sometimes walk miles to the school. Seventy-five dollars a month here is about the same as a teacher starting out in Vancouver would get. Half of that or more goes for room and board in either case. Of course we get our uniforms, and have them laundered. Do you know you'll be paying three per cent income tax? But it's better than no work, no money."

I knew about no work, no money. People were just beginning to realize in the early 1930's that 'times were tight' though we couldn't know that the Depression would last for ten years. It had become increasingly difficult to find employment. Later figures showed that in 1933 over 800,000 Canadians out of a total work force of four and a quarter million were unemployed. Tens of thousands of young men had never held a job. There was no unemployment insurance. Federal relief camps had been opened in 1932 to provide food and shelter, paying 20 cents a day to 20,000 men. Soup kitchens fed many who tramped the streets, sleeping in parks or under bridges at night. Economic distress was very real.

The dayroom workers were gathering at the rotunda door, their work finished. "You can take them out to the utility room, Lehman," Richmond said. "No, not the floor polishers. They may carry on all afternoon, too. It's a real compulsion with them."

Seated again in the dayroom, I observed the strange facial and vocal expressions and the many variations of bizarre behavior with bemused interest. Grimaces and fidgeting were outward signs of inner disturbance, sometimes manifested by a shout or a groan, or a fist raised against an unseen enemy. Obsessed remarks indicating inner torment were shouted repeatedly. A small, thin woman dressed in the blue broadcloth ward dress that most of the women wore, suddenly sprang from her chair shouting, "No, no! Don't take it away! Oh, God, it's floating away!" She reached frantically into the air, then subsided into her chair sobbing quietly.

A distracted woman passed on an endless circuit of the room. "All gone to water. I've all gone to water. That's all I am, just water." Her voice trailed off, to be heard again on her next ceaseless round.

A woman approached making strange little jumps that had a definite pattern. Three steps and a jump, three steps and a jump. Richmond explained, "She thinks there are electric wires she has to hop over, or she'll be electrocuted. Electricity is a new concept to many of the older women and they get strange fixations about it."

"I can understand that," I admitted. "When I first heard a radio, I looked behind it to see where the man was who was talking. I was pretty young," I added sheepishly.

We hadn't been sitting long when the office door opened and a tall, solidly-built man with a dominating presence, wearing a doctor's white coat, entered. He was accompanied by Miss Hicks, Superintendent of Nurses, and Miss Marlatt. Miss Coghlan was the fourth person of this distinguished group, ready to answer questions and report on patients. Richmond rose and I followed her example. " Dr. Ryan," she murmured, "makes rounds every morning."

At the end of the room Queenie was bristling, ready to do battle as Dr. Ryan approached. She swore and called him 'son-of-a-bitch' and 'filthy swine', and other choice epithets which he ignored as he slowly scanned the patients in turn, stopping to ask a question now and then but passing Queenie without comment. "She believes Dr. Ryan is responsible for her being here," Richmond explained. "This goes on every morning."

As the party passed us to move on into the second dayroom, Dr. Ryan nodded to Richmond and subjected me to a searching look that had me inwardly squirming. "I feel like I've been under a microscope," I said when they were out of hearing.

"I'm positive he assesses the nurses as well as the patients," Richmond chuckled. "A perfect example of gimlet eyes."

Not long after rounds were finished Gladwin brought back her dormitory workers and Richmond left us, saying, "I'll help Dawson put the linens away or whatever needs to be finished."

"What's dormitory duty like?" I asked curiously. "Are you all finished there?"

Gladwin settled down in the chair beside me. "It's easy. The women know what to do. They get their cleaning stuff and they go right ahead on their own. The only thing is, they're not very good at making square corners, so you spend most of your time re-doing the corners on 100 beds. Miss Hicks is really strict about square corners; she'll pull a sloppy one right out and have you do it over. They inspect the dormitories sometimes, you know, especially when there's someone in bed for the day."

"Sick, you mean? Do we have to take care of them in bed?"

"Just for something temporary, like a bad cold. There is an Infirmary..."

"Where? In this building?" I was trying to get a picture of the wards in my mind; I dreaded turning the wrong way and getting lost, on my own.

"Right above the patients' dining room and the kitchens. And Ward J is above that, you may as well know. That's the cell ward. It has 40 side-rooms - that's what we call the cells."

I shuddered. Surely they wouldn't place a probationer on the cell ward. "Well, dormitory duty sounds OK," I said, "if that's all you do."

"Well, not all," Gladwin admitted. "We have to clean the black marks off the floors. We have to use strong ammonia gel - it's made up here - that can't be in the patients' hands. Black marks are never-ending. They're compressed wax where the legs of the beds rub on the floor, so you finish the whole dorm - it takes days - then start over again. But nobody stands over you to see how fast you do them, and if you weren't doing that you'd be cleaning brass door knobs or washing windows. The dinner buzzer will be going in a few minutes. We'd better start rounding up the laggards."

In the afternoon Gladwin and I were given the job of rubbing the black marks off the dormitory floors. We picked up the ammonia cleaner from the locked utility room. "Smell that," Gladwin said, prying the lid off the tin. "Not too close," she warned. "The first time I was given this job, I was told to just smell the tins as I opened them, and I'd know which one was ammonia. It's unmarked because it's made here. So I took the lid off and put the tin right up to my nose and drew in a breath, and it almost took the top of my head off. My eyes ran and my nose stung, and it was hours before I felt right again."

The dormitory space was as extensive as the dayrooms, but divided into smaller rooms with a washroom at the corner of the two main corridors, and a shower room. The showers, like the toilet stalls, had no doors. "They must have figured the nurses need supervision in the showers, like the patients," I remarked. "I noticed last night there aren't any doors in our showers in the Nurses' Home, either."

"Thank goodness there are tub compartments for us, complete with doors," Gladwin said. She and I had both chosen a tub bath. "You get used to nudity, a certain amount, but it's not my cup of tea." I fervently agreed.

"Imagine being on night duty here," Gladwin said. "All lights are out, even in the corridors, except for one gooseneck lamp over the nurses' table and a blue light in each dormitory room." Besides the windows on the outer walls, the rooms were lined with the same small-paned windows along the corridors so that beds could be seen from the halls.

"Where's the nurses' table?" I asked. The corridors were bare of furniture.

"They bring one in from the rotunda," Gladwin said. "And two easy chairs. One nurse sits with her back to one corridor and the other one with her back to the other corridor." It sounded terribly spooky, and dangerous.

We were on our knees rubbing at the detested spots at the base of each bedpost. "Four hundred bedposts," I muttered. "No wonder it's a never-ending job. I'd rather wash windows or polish door knobs."

"Richmond has those all figured out, too," Gladwin said. "She said there are 47,440 window panes in this building, 452 doors, two knobs to a door. She is a stickler for detail."

The afternoon passed pleasantly, and as we chatted our friendship grew. There were no coffee breaks in the early 30's and only young knees could endure the constant squatting or kneeling required. Being called back to the dayroom for supper hour was a relief.

By the end of the long day I was tired, mentally and physically. I had absorbed much that was new and strange, but I was far easier in my mind than I had been that morning, and I could smile at my wild imaginings. Short as our mealtimes were, the light-hearted conversation was refreshing. Though Fraser's gloominess persisted, it was disregarded.

Humorous incidents were shared. Langley told a story on herself as she walked back to the Nurses' Home with Gladwin and me:

They were just going out the front door with a group of women, taking them for a walk, and she was at the end of the line. She saw a woman coming out of the reception room so she took her by the sleeve and said, 'Come on. Out this way.'

"She pulled away and looked at me as if I was crazy. 'I'm just going to visit my sister. What did you think I was doing?' Was my face red!"

We were laughing as we entered the Nurses' Home. Was it only 24 hours since I had first come in this door? My thoughts went back to my introduction to the Home and my first meeting with some of the fun-loving girls who would make working in a mental hospital not only bearable but a fascinating experience.

Raised on a farm in the Fraser Valley, thwarted in my plans to go to university by the economic depression, I faced a totally foreign experience, not at all confident that I would be able to endure the situation. On my first visit my heart beat had quickened as the bus slowed down for the Nurses' Home after passing the threatening buildings of the Provincial Mental Hospital. I had now entered one and found it to be as normal as a daily routine of ordinary occupations could make it.

Checking in at the Nurses' Home last night had been scary but turned out to be an introduction to the light-hearted side of my new life. My thoughts went back to that moment.

CHAPTER TWO

The Greyhound bus came to a stop at the walk that led to the front door of the Nurses' Home. I saw a long white building, two-storied except for the section above the entrance located near one end, which had an extra story, its gable end facing the street. Gripping my suitcase tightly, I went up the walk and apprehensively pressed the bell.

The door was opened by a girl in bathrobe and slippers, her hair set in waves held flat by rows of bobby pins. She noted my suitcase and my air of uncertainty and opened the door wide. "Another probie, right? Come in. I'll look up Miss Whitehorse. Just wait here," and she ran off through French doors on my left that led into a comfortably furnished living room. She disappeared through the first of two doors on the right of it.

I was standing in a square hall at the center of a continual movement of traffic, in and out of the living room, up and down the stairs in the left corner of the hall, along the corridor on my right that stretched the length of the building with rooms on either side.

There were girls everywhere. Some were still in uniform; others had changed into pajamas and robes. They took scant notice of me as they chattered in groups of two or three, or hurried through the living room to the door at the end, pulling a pack of cigarettes out of a pocket on the way.

A radio was blaring somewhere, and a piano was being idly plinked not far from where I stood. Two nurses rushed in the front door, one exclaiming breathlessly, "Wouldn't you know the count would be off the very first time I have a date with Gary! He said 7:30 and it's almost that now!" She dashed up the stairs ahead of her companion, almost colliding with two girls coming down, dressed for town and carrying suitcases. "We'll just make the bus! Hurry!"

I heard as they ran out the front door.

A phone shrilled loudly and one of the girls passing through turned aside to a cubby-hole under the stairs to answer it. She came to the bottom of the stairs and yelled, "Royston!" in a voice that would carry to the farthest room, then went up the stairs, dodging an impetuous girl who came hurtling down to the phone. I could hear her conversation clearly.

"Hello? Oh, Mother." The drop in inflection revealed disappointment. "I'm fine. I'll be home Monday night. Yeah, two days off. I'll tell you all about it when I get home. No, not bad at all. You get used to it. Even getting up at six o'clock in the morning! See you Monday." She hung up and tore back up the stairs two at a time.

A harassed looking elderly nurse with her sparse white hair twisted into a knot on which a high white cap perched precariously, hurried in from the living room, complaining, "No sense of responsibility! They think I'm paid to clean up after them!" She consulted a paper on the desk and turned to me, fixing me with a disapproving stare as she said, "Miss Lehman? Follow me." She started up the stairs ahead of me, her querulous voice going on without pause. "Someone let soup boil over in the kitchen and I had to wait to see who came for it so I could make her clean it up. Why girls on nights don't go over for supper is beyond me."

We had turned at the landing and were now at the second floor where Miss Whitehorse turned again to the next flight of stairs. She continued peevishly, "So much to do. Such thoughtless girls. No consideration at all. It was different in my day. We didn't have a smoking room, for one thing. Those girls will burn the place down one of these days."

At the second landing she stopped suddenly and shot me a suspicious look. "You're not to sleep together! Do you hear?" She was actually quivering as she spoke, and she bristled with malevolent indignation as she pressed her thin lips together and went up the last few steps in brooding silence.

What could she mean? Sisters slept together, brothers slept together, friends slept with you when they visited. I couldn't imagine anything wrong with it, but I hated the implication of wrong-doing and at that moment I hated Miss Whitehorse for suggesting it.

Now on the third floor, we passed a row of lockers in a short hall that led to the dormitory. This room stretched from the front to the back of the Home, with four beds along each wall, a dresser and wooden straight chair by each bed. A set of large windows in each gable end was covered with thin curtains that blew gently inward in a light breeze. Drapes at the sides were pulled back to let in the fresh air. There were two wash basins in one corner.

Half a dozen girls stopped what they were doing when we came in and faced Miss Whitehorse warily. She pounced immediately.

"Miss Dunbar! Put on a robe, at once!" She was shaking with outrage as she spit out the words. "I've told you the boys stand on the bank behind the Home looking in! Pull the drapes closed when you're changing! It's indecent the way you run around practically naked." The last word was uttered as an imprecation.

The target of this attack was a pretty girl with soft skin now flushed a rosy red, wearing brief panties and a bra, who had been washing her white stockings and some undies at one of the basins. Her figure was perfect. Anyone with that figure would want to show it off, I thought. She pulled on a dressing gown, her face mutinous.

Satisfied but still venomous, Miss Whitehorse turned to me and led me to the one bed that was unmade, with the bedding neatly piled up on one end. "You'll have this bed." She shot a suspicious glance around at the girls and asked, "Why is it always the one by the fire escape?" Without waiting for an answer as six faces stared back at her in blank innocence, she continued her instructions to me.

"This is the key to your locker; the number is on the key. Keep it locked. The dormitory is cleaned by patients, but you're to keep it tidy. Bed made, clothes put away. Nothing of value left around; that's what lockers are for." There was a stir of laughter and Miss Whitehorse glowered, her expression one of sourness and irritation.

"When you've unpacked and made up your bed, come down and get your uniform and your key. For the wards," she explained impatiently at my bewildered look. "You have to sign for the key. And you're not to take it home, or off the grounds! Put it in your locker on your days off." With a last virulent glance at Dunbar, Miss Whitehorse bustled out.

"Whew! She gets worse, I think, with each new probie. I wonder why she hates us so much? Did she give you that line about not sleeping together? As if anyone'd want to sleep two to one of these beds!" Dunbar's nose wrinkled in scorn. "A nice welcome we all get from our housemother," with heavy emphasis on the last word. She had thrown off her robe the minute Miss Whitehorse left - the sleeves were wide and interfered with her washing - and was back at the basin. She rinsed out her undies with a wicked gleam in her eyes. "Silly old bat! Her name should be 'Warhorse.' I know what will make her lose her teeth!" She opened the drapes that had been closed at Miss Whitehorse's bidding, and pinned her panties to the sheers.

The girls laughed and resumed their nightly routine, washing clothes, cleaning white shoes, shampooing and setting hair, and pinning collars and cuffs on fresh blue uniforms. I had my suitcase open and was deciding where to put things when a sturdily-built girl flopped onto my bed. Her straight brown hair was so short it was almost a boyish cut, but she had a spit-curl at one side of her square forehead which softened the effect. She had changed to outdoor clothes. Her friendly face was free of make-up, having a healthy glow of its own.

"Name's Gladwin," she offered. "When you're all put away I'll help you make your bed." She stretched out comfortably with her head on my pillows.

"My name is Eva," I began, but was interrupted with, "We don't use our first names, Lehman. That's what Whitey said your name was, didn't she? She sure gets wound up. She's going to blow a fuse one day. I kind of feel sorry for her. She's too old to be in a place like this." Dunbar was within earshot and gave a rude raspberry. "Whitey Hee-Haw never was young," she hooted.

Gladwin grinned. "Now you know very well that you get a kick out of riling her, Dunbar. Look at those panties on the curtains! What's going to happen is that you'll go down for a smoke, and one of us will end up getting the blast from Whitehorse." Gladwin started to help me make the bed.

"Oh, jeeze. I guess so. Down they come." Dunbar hung the panties on her towel rod and went out, wearing her robe.

"Dunbar's not a bad sort," Gladwin said. "In fact I haven't met a bad egg yet, and I've been here a couple of weeks."

"Why does everyone use last names? It seems funny to be called Lehman. Can't you call me Eva?"

"Nope, sorry. It's because I might forget on the wards and the patients would pick up on it, and you'd lose authority. See?" Gladwin was carefully making hospital corners on her side of the bed, and she looked at the carelessly tucked in sheets on my side. "Hey, I'd better show you how to make square corners. This dorm's inspected once in awhile - Miss Hicks and Miss Marlatt have rooms at the bottom of the stairs here on the second floor, and they can come up anytime. Miss Hicks is very particular about square corners." I thought of the immaculate Superintendent of Nurses, who had interviewed me for the job. Meticulous she would certainly be.

My bed made and my suitcase stored in my locker, I looked around. I recognized Royston from the phone call, although her head was wrapped in a towel after a shampoo. Gladwin was stretched out on her own bed next to mine.

Royston was staring moodily at her reflection in her dresser mirror. "I've washed my hair and forgot Langley's off to set it. Darn, I can't get the waves pinned the way she does it." She was jabbing bobby pins aimlessly at the waves she was forming with her fingers.

"Here, Royston. You wave and I'll put in the pins." A short dark girl came up behind Royston's chair and started competently putting pins in the waves. An expression of serenity distinguished this straight-backed girl whose shoulders were unnaturally rigid like those of soldiers on parade. Determination showed in the lines of her body and the set of her lips, but there was a glint of laughter in her soft brown eyes.

"You'll be doing Langley out of her job as the dormitory hairdresser, Oliver," Gladwin said, running a comb through her short bob. "That's one thing I don't have to worry about, is setting my hair. Yours looks like a natural wave, Lehman. Langley will be the next one to move downstairs to a room; she and Kelsey are the seniors in the dorm now."

"Seniors?" I was puzzled. " I thought there were just probationers in the dormitory."

"There are." A discontented-looking girl whose heavy dark bangs shaded her eyes had drifted over. "We're all probies," she said, "but everyone is senior or junior to everyone else. It's not like classes that all start at the same time. Miss Hicks has been taking on new girls every other day for the past month, but never two at the same time. So I'm senior to Gladwin but junior to Royston. Come on, Glad," she said abruptly. "You promised you'd go for a walk with me. Are you coming?" She absent-mindedly picked at a pimple on her chin.

"OK, keep your shirt on, Fraser. I'm ready. Want to come with us, Lehman?"

"I'd better not. I have to go down for my uniform and get things lined up for the morning." Where had I put my white shoes and stockings? The two girls went out.

Royston remarked, "I don't think Fraser will be with us very much longer. Have you heard her say she's thinking of getting married? Just to get out of here? She's not that struck on the boyfriend."

"She's foolish to marry him then," Oliver stated firmly.

"Well, there aren't any other jobs to go to," said Royston. "I know. I looked for nearly a year after I finished school."

"Me, too," I said. I thought of that hopeless search, answering ads only to find someone ahead of me, already hired. I had gone into every store in New Westminster, filling out application forms in some, seeing all the other unemployed doing the same thing. There wasn't even housework to be had, and I would have gladly done that type of work just to make a dollar. My father had been caught in the Great Depression, though nobody called it that at the beginning of the 1930's, but when it went on for over ten years until war-related jobs opened up in the 1940's, then the 1930's became known, deservedly, as the 'Dirty Thirties'.

Hadn't Miss Hicks told me, when I filled in the application form for psychiatric nurse's training, that there were 200 ahead of me? I was lucky to get this job.

That thought and the satisfaction I would get in wearing a nurse's uniform cheered me as I waited for Miss Whitehorse in the downstairs hall. I could hear her scolding voice in the smoking room, and the wave of laughter that arose after she bustled out. She flushed when she saw me and realizing I had heard, spoke angrily. "Always somebody wanting something. Think I'm paid to wait on them," and she pinched her lips together in their customary downward curve.

Impatiently she piled the uniform pieces into my arms. Blue uniform dress, white starched apron, bib, collar, cuffs, a wide starched belt, and a strong leather belt with the heavy key on a metal ring attached to it by means of a leather strap. Then she pulled a book out of the desk for me to sign for the key, and I had to unload it all to hold the pen, unfortunately giggling while I did so. The very sight of me seemed to annoy her anyway, and she rounded on me sharply.

"That's enough! Mind your manners! Now you're responsible for that key, and you're to leave it in your locker on your days off. Do you understand? You're not to take it home."

I was glad to escape back to the dorm. Royston was writing a letter while her hair dried and Oliver was propped on her pillows reading a book. "Back from the war?" she asked, her eyes dancing though she kept a straight face.

I was quickly beginning to feel very comfortable with these girls. Even Fraser, unhappy as she appeared to be, had an appeal, perhaps because she was agonizing between two situations, work or marriage, neither of which she really wanted. Gladwin had been helpful, probably because my bed was right next to hers, and she had an honesty and innate dignity about her that I admired. Living in the dormitory was going to be interesting.

When Gladwin returned she took me down to the second floor washrooms. One was a lavatory with a row of toilet cubicles and hand-basins. The other room had four showers and two tubs. I was shocked to see that the shower stalls had no doors, but a couple of girls were showering unconcernedly, apparently not at all shy about their bodies. Gladwin and I retreated to the privacy of the tubs, each of which was in its own compartment with a door.

Passing the lockers on the way back to the dormitory, Gladwin chuckled. "Miss Whitehorse may believe you need to match your key number to the locker, but we found that any even-numbered key will open all even-numbered lockers, and so with the odd numbers."

"Nobody has anything expensive so it doesn't matter much," Fraser added. "Our $33 a month won't buy furs or jewelry, or even a radio."

"A few of the senior nurses have radios, so maybe we'll be able to afford one some day. If we stay long enough," Dunbar chimed in, back from her smoke downstairs.

Fraser muttered, "Well, I won't," and got into bed.

"My dentist will get a big chunk of my money," I said. "Before I was eight, I had to have my front teeth straightened, but there wasn't room to bring this one forward." I tapped the tooth that was in behind the others, giving me a gap-toothed appearance unless you looked closely. "I'm going to get that one pulled and a peg tooth in there," I vowed. "And the fillings I always need! I've had too much of that horrible drill. The dentist who figured out how to straighten my teeth used to put that drill on and he didn't stop until he had the hole drilled out ready for a filling. Pure torture!" I shuddered. That was before cocaine was in general use as a dental anesthetic.

"You're lucky you were sent to the dentist at all," said Gladwin, whose front teeth were slightly crowded. " How did he straighten them, and what did it cost?"

"He put long gold covers over these three, see?" I indicated the teeth that had been brought forward. "All four of them were behind the bottom teeth - I must have looked like a bull-dog. Then I must have looked queer all those months with the gold, twice as long as the teeth underneath. But the dentist called me 'the girl with the golden smile' and that made me kind of proud. Anyway the gold made the bottom teeth move back where they should have been, and gradually forced the top teeth forward. When he took off the gold covers, my bite was corrected - except for this." I tapped the offending tooth with distaste.

Gladwin started to speak and I hastily added, "Oh, yes. It cost eight dollars."

The girls had all been listening and there was a buzz of conversation about dental problems. They all knew that dental work was extremely painful, and cost too much.

Langley came in from her day off, a tall friendly girl with straight dark hair worn in a long bob almost to her shoulders. She talked vivaciously about what she had done at home, and her hair swung around with her quick movements as she unpacked.

"Does someone have an alarm clock?" I asked. "How do we wake up in time in the morning?"

"You'll hear the bell!" Fraser said. "Miss Whitehorse comes past all the rooms with a hand-bell, like we used to have at school. I think she enjoys waking us up. She knows we'd like to sleep later. Six o'clock is too darned early to get up. And 12 hours is too long a workday," she added, voicing some of the gripes she had about the job. She picked at a hang-nail, then bit it off.

"Ten-thirty. Lights out," Oliver looked to see that everyone was settled, then flicked the switch. The dormitory became silent.

The fears that had beset me since I'd heard I was hired came back in full force as I turned this way and that in the strange bed, tormented by ideas of insane behavior. Then a new worry entered my mind. What if an inmate escaped in the night and came up the fire-escape and landed on my bed? So that was why this bed was always left for the newest girl!

The quiet breathing around me at last convinced me that these girls, who had been on the wards, were not lying awake worrying, and I drifted off to sleep.

I was awakened by a foot, then a shadowy person landing on my bed, and I knew my worst fears had come true. I tried to scream but my throat was tight and dry. "Sh-h-h! It's me. Sullivan. My boyfriend gave me a boost up the fire-escape. I'm sort of late." She giggled. "Can I leave my shoes under your bed? I'll get them tomorrow." She crept out in her stocking feet, going down the stairs to her room.

Why, oh why had I ever come to this place? In a few hours I would be amongst the insane. Unable to go back to sleep, my troubled mind churned over the events of the past week. How quickly my life had changed!

CHAPTER THREE

Essondale! called the bus driver. My heart jolted painfully. This was where I would get off, to be interviewed for a position at the Provincial Mental Hospital, the center of psychiatric care in the 1930's and for decades to come. Insane people unable to live normal lives were brought here from all over the province to be kept under lock and key.

We had turned off the main road about five miles out of New Westminster and were winding up a wide avenue toward the jail-like buildings lined up on a terrace halfway up the gentle slope. On either side of us as we drove through the grounds were green lawns shaded by a variety of trees - maples, oaks and elms interspersed with tall pyramidal or grandly-spreading evergreens that flourished in our Pacific Coast climate. Flowering ornamental cherry trees and graceful magnolias celebrated spring with a profusion of pastel-colored blossoms, completing a vision of well-planned beauty.

The bus stopped in front of the middle red brick building brooding over the peaceful valley below. Half-a-dozen passengers alighted and disappeared purposefully. Full of misgivings, I stepped off after them. Working here was far removed from my dreams of further education but I could not go on living idly at home. Jobs in the 1930's were scarce, almost non-existent, and I would like to earn some money. But this kind of work, amongst the insane, had never entered my mind until my mother saw the advertisement.

"They have a training course for psychiatric nursing, Eva. You could try it. You don't have to stay if you don't like it." My mother had seen my disappointment at not finding something to do. So here I was, half hoping I wouldn't be taken on.

While this was going through my mind I was studying the forbidding buildings. Each had numerous wings lined with closely-barred windows branching out from a central section, with an imposing entrance framed with white pillars a full two stories high. There were three main stories plus an attic with dormer windows, and a basement section, painted white. All the windows were made up of small square panes which created the barred appearance and would certainly prevent escape by that means. It was a somber institution.

Putting off the moment when I would have to keep my appointment with the Superintendent of Nurses, I looked back the way I had come. Rich farmlands bordered the meandering Coquitlam River all the way to its junction with the wide waterway that was nearly at the end of its long and turbulent journey from the Rocky Mountains to the Pacific Ocean. Here, on the last stretch through the flatlands created in the years before dykes were built to control its floodings, the Fraser River was peaceful and subdued, subject only to the ebb and flow of the ocean's tides.

I was looking down at nearly six hundred acres of Colony Farm, a subsidiary of the hospital institution and a source of much of the food required by its population of nearly three thousand inmates and several hundred staff. Besides the large barns there was one institutional-type square building for patients and some smaller housing for the attendants. The farm workers preferred this life in the outdoors to incarceration up on the hill.

There was also housing for attendants and maintenance staff on the hillside behind these three buildings where I stood, I learned later. But now, though fearful of setting foot inside, procrastination must end. I knew I could not put off keeping my appointment any longer.

The only persons in sight were two men in loose, nondescript pants and shirts who sat on a bench nearby. I hesitatingly approached and asked if they could tell me which was the Female Chronic building. One averted his face and kept his head down, but the other rose to his lanky six-foot length and loquaciously told me more than I had expected to hear.

"That's it over there, the last one. Just opened a couple years ago for the screeching women. We were glad to get rid of them outta here, though there's a women's admitting ward in this middle building still. Say, are you looking to be a nurse here?" He leered. "I'll give you a tip, now. When you get to live in the Nurses' Home - that's farther along down the hill a bit, past those doctor's houses - don't hang your pretty undies on the clothesline at the back. This fellow here sneaks over and swipes them. Don't you, Herbie? Got some on now?" He leered suggestively.

They were inmates! Hurriedly I backed away, thanking my informant who was grinning widely, and started toward the women's building. A sidewalk extended along the edge of the avenue that wound past the buildings, and widened into a parking space in front of each building. It now became evident that there was a porch at the end of each wing at both sides of the center section, for the barred squares there were without glass. A woman had climbed onto an inside sill and was wailing loudly as she clung to the bars that imprisoned her. Other figures could be seen pacing about, and the confused sounds they made suggested tormented souls facing irrational fears and undescribable terrors. Noisy seagulls swooped around and clustered at an open section of window where somebody inside was feeding bread to them. Their hoarse cries were fitting accompaniment to the fears that were slowing my steps.

Struggling to suppress a surge of fright, I climbed the impressively wide granite steps that swept up to a colonnaded porch. Double doors surmounted by a stained-glass transom stood open.

My steps faltered. Just then two young nurses in all-white uniforms came out, talking and laughing, and ran down the steps. Their cheerfulness was comforting. If they could work here, it must be bearable. And how attractive that uniform was! I took a deep breath and went in.

The gleaming entrance hall was lined with administrative offices and led to an Information desk by the elevator at the far end. The pleasant middle-aged man at the desk was greeting me when a light began flashing on a telephone exchange board by his side. He turned to answer it.

"Miss Marlatt? One moment, please." The connection was no sooner made than another light went on. This call brought a frenzy of action. Rapidly plugging into one line after another, the man said urgently into each one, "Help on J! Help on J!" and repeated it for about six calls.

My imagination was fired with visions of the violence that would require such a summons and my spirits sank again. But there was no turning back now, as I was directed to the office where I would be interviewed by the Superintendent of Nurses.

"Miss Hicks? Is she expecting you? Fine. It's the second door on the left." I knocked timidly on the open door.

Miss Constance Alberta Hicks sat behind a large desk that would have overwhelmed her small figure had she not sat so straight. Dark eyes bright with vitality examined me closely. Her face was framed by dark hair carefully waved, on which a high white nurse's cap was perched. There was something bird-like about her, a suggestion of quick reactions, of being in control of herself and her surroundings. Her crisp uniform was spotless.

"Miss Lehman?" she said briskly. "Sit down, please. Why do you want to work here?"

The question was unexpected, and considering my conflicting feelings, almost unanswerable. I stammered something about having looked for work since I finished High School and finding nothing.

"We have a three-year nursing program here," Miss Hicks announced, her observant eyes noting my confusion and doubt. "The lectures start in the fall and they cover the same subjects as in general nursing with the addition of psychiatry. You would have to study, as well as work a 12-hour day. Are you prepared to do that?"

My interest had been caught and I relaxed. I was not intimidated by study - I had studied Senior Matriculation subjects along with two other High School graduates out in the country before our family moved into New Westminster. Then I joined the class at the Duke of Connaught High School and finished the last four months successfully. I welcomed the opportunity to get a nursing education. I'd like that, I answered briefly.

"Fill out this application form, then, but I have to warn you that there are 200 ahead of you." She smiled kindly though her words were discouraging. I took the form into a reception room by the front door as she returned to the papers on her desk.

This form was like many others I had seen and I concentrated on suitable answers. Date - April 8, 1933. Name - Eva Lehman.

Date of birth... I paused. In four months I would be 17, surely too young to be accepted. I could put back the year of my birth by one year, and I still might be judged too young. Nurses usually started at 18 so I had better add two years to my actual age of 16. After all, I had gone through High School with students two years older than I and got along fine with them. That morning I had drawn my shoulder-length hair back and pinned it in a soft roll to make me look older. Resolutely I put down the false date.

I had just written 4th year High after Education when I was interrupted. A girl had come in shortly after me with a similar form and was seated opposite me at the table. Now she asked, "What did you put for Education?"

I looked up. Bold eyes in an aggressive face stared audaciously at me. Her chin was thrust defiantly forward, her dark hair combed back carelessly off her forehead.

"Fourth year High," I answered. In our province at that time High School was completed in three years, with a Junior Matriculation certificate. The fourth year was the equivalent of the first year of university, and students with a Senior Matriculation standing were accepted into the second year of university.

"Well I'm putting 4th year too," she said, tossing her head defiantly. "I repeated second year and I'm in 3rd year now so that's four years, near enough." She began writing again.

Of all the nerve, I fumed inwardly, conveniently forgetting the adjustment of my birth date. I know, I'll put in 'Sr. Matric.' There's room. And I have the certificate to prove it.

We finished our papers together, prevaricators both, and handed them over to Miss Hicks, who said merely, "I'll phone if there's an opening."

"Not much chance," I said to Sara Renfrew after we had exchanged names on the way out. "Did she tell you there were 200 ahead of you?"

"Yeah, but a friend of mine got on a few weeks ago and she says you have a good chance if you have Senior Matric. I hear the lectures are tough."

Maybe she was only looking for summer work, I mused after we parted. She didn't sound like much of a scholar.

The phone call the next day was a complete surprise. "Miss Hicks speaking. I'd like you to start on Monday. Can you report to the Nurses' Home early Sunday evening? And come out tomorrow to be measured for uniforms." It was a statement rather than a question. I accepted, my heart beating madly.

Being measured for uniforms proved to be my introduction to the Occupational Therapy department which spread over a large part of the attic floor. Miss Hicks began instructing me in correct terminology in the elevator. "We call the inmates 'patients', and they are mentally ill, not insane," she stated briskly. "Essondale is one of the finest and best equipped mental hospitals on the North American continent, and our nursing program one of the most advanced." There was justifiable pride in her voice, for I learned that it was Miss Hicks who initiated the program when this building was opened a few years previously.

The elevator opened into a small room with locked doors on each side. Miss Hicks unlocked the one to the right, and I realized when that door clanged shut behind us that I was locked into this dreadful place and had no means to get myself out. I stayed close to Miss Hicks as we passed small rooms fitted into the double or triple dormer windows.

Miss Hicks pointed out a beauty parlor, equipped as well as any in the city. All the usual procedures were in progress: shampoos, cuts, marcels, finger-waving. Dryers were whirring and women were sitting along the wall waiting for their turn. "Most of the patients have their hair trimmed by a barber who visits the wards, but those who wish may have their hair done here, when they can get an appointment. It's a busy place," Miss Hicks explained.

We were passing rooms equipped with craft materials of all kinds. An older woman in a white uniform dress looked up and smiled at us, then went on with the help she was giving a young woman who was painstakingly weaving at a loom. "Miss Duncan is our Occupational Therapist," Miss Hicks continued, "this is an important part of our treatment of the mentally ill. Having something useful to do gives them a feeling of accomplishment and aids in their recovery. It provides them with familiar tasks or teaches them new skills."

The Superintendent of Nurses now opened a door to our right and we entered the busiest room of all, where the sewing and mending were done. Several women were at treadle sewing machines which were whirring busily. Others were sewing on buttons, or doing hand mending. A few poor souls were seated on the floor apathetically pulling apart knitted garments and winding the wool into untidy balls. A harried-looking woman in a white uniform came from the far end of the large room where patients were doing touch-up ironing or folding clean laundry, placing it into compartments along the wall. "This is Miss Lehman, a new probationer, Mrs. Rupert," said Miss Hicks, and she went off to circle the room, stopping now and then to talk to a patient.

Mrs. Rupert produced a tape measure and began taking my measurements, fretting all the while. "So many new nurses this time of year," she said as she marked down the figures. "And a set of three uniforms to make for each one. As well as the regular work, patients' dresses and shifts, their sheets and pillow cases, and all the mending, and the hand-ironing the laundry can't do. And these women are so unreliable. There's one going off now." I had heard a loud muttering from one of the women at a sewing machine, and her handling of the garment she was working on was agitated and rough. "I don't know why they brought her up from the ward, I'll have to phone them to come and get her. And those two quarreling over there are always at it. Just can't abide each other. I start them well apart but they gravitate together every time. If I had some help...There's enough work for two or three supervisors here. But I have to handle it all myself."

Miss Hicks had come up and heard this complaint. "And you're doing a fine job, Mrs. Rupert. Will you have those uniforms over at the Nurses Home by Friday?" Miss Hicks' request was obviously an order, for Mrs. Rupert's grumblings ceased abruptly, yet she managed to convey her sense of overwork by answering, "Well, I'll get one of everything done somehow. The rest can wait until next week. You can pick them up then, Miss Lehman, when the nurses come in for their clean uniforms." We left her hurrying over to the two fractious women whose voices had been rising, while she cast anxious glances at the agitated woman at the sewing machine.

Miss Hicks gave me final instructions in her office. "You provide your own white stockings, and white shoes. Get sensible nurses' oxfords. And you'll need studs for the belt, and lots of safety pins. Sturdy ones," she smiled. With a short explanation of the days off, seven per month - "It works out to working four days and one off, or sometimes two days off together and you work longer in between" - she dismissed me.

Though I began the work with much trepidation, the three years I would spend in a mental hospital proved to be exciting, challenging, and certainly educational. The few bad moments were offset by the many benefits. The nursing course was invaluable, and wearing a nurses' uniform was a constant pleasure. Living with more than 100 young women was an education in itself, and lifelong friendships were formed.

I learned to be tolerant of the unfortunates who cannot cope with reality and who become dependent on institutional care. Many patients were simply senile, many others appeared to be as normal as anyone 'outside' when not seized by the frenzy of psychotic disorders. A few were suffering from epilepsy, at that time considered a certifiable condition. Before the discovery of more sophisticated drugs and treatments, very few patients were released to normal living.

As a result the mental hospitals of that era must ever expand to accommodate the increasing numbers of patients. We were told in our lectures that one person in ten would spend some part of his or her life in a psychiatric institution. In a literal sense I have served my time; but, fortunately for me, I carried a key.

CHAPTER FOUR

Once the first day was safely over I was able to relax. My previous notions of an 'insane asylum' were so far from the truth, at least on ward H2, they appeared ridiculous in retrospect. I was now looking forward to each day with relish. There was so much to learn.

A morning with Gladwin in the dormitories enabled me to anticipate handling that assignment on my own. It also served as an introduction to some of the better patients, who accomplished their accustomed tasks capably and contentedly. Working closely with them produced a friendly relationship that made the hours pass quickly. In spite of Gladwin's admonitions about unpredictable, unstable personalities, I could not envision these apparently normal women becoming agitated - 'possessed with the devil' - as Mrs. Ridley had been. She was now subdued by sedatives to a stuporous calmness, and in time would be back to a more reasonable state - until the next frenzy.

Careful attention to the standards set by the Superintendent of Nurses kept us fully occupied. The beds must be lined up just so, evenly spaced. Pillows must be placed in the exact center of the bed, ends tucked in and facing away from the door. "When there's someone in bed, like Mrs. Ridley when she was heavily sedated, she has to be in the exact center of the bed for the doctor's morning visit," Gladwin said seriously. Was she pulling my leg, I wondered? But she went on, "That's when Miss Hicks checks our work. You'd better learn to make square corners to suit her, Lehman. She'll rip them out and make you do them over if they don't look neat enough."

Ever ready to quibble, I put forth a weak argument. "How can they be square corners when they're triangular when they're finished? And you use triangles to make them, too."

"Oh, Lehman!" Gladwin was laughing, but exasperated. "What difference does it make what they're called! Watch, now. Start by pulling the bottom sheet tight, under the mattress..." She went through the steps one by one, and I decided I had better master the art of making hospital corners. So automatic did they become that I make 'square corners' on my beds to this day.

The idea of night duty haunted me. They were on duty 12 hours too, coming on when we left at seven and there until seven in the morning. "How do they stay awake?" I asked Gladwin.

"Oh, the night staff supervise bedtime, and showers. And they get the women up and dressed and into the dayrooms in the morning. They get off for a midnight meal, too - just the one break. And there's a doctor making rounds, and the Night Supervisor."

"How long are the night shifts? How many months, I mean?"

"Anywhere from four to six months, or more sometimes. I think we'd better get the ladies together and go back to the dayrooms. The buzzer will be going for dinner, soon. Anything not done can wait until this afternoon."

On another day I accompanied Dawson on her errands. The patients were always taken by the wide cement stairways located off the rotunda and at the entrance to the ward, opposite the dining room. We took Occupational Therapy workers up two floors to the attic, and dropped off the ones with appointments at the beauty parlor. We could leave them there and pick them up later, but had to stay with anyone taken over to the Acute Building for a doctor's or dentist's appointment. The dental equipment was as good or better than any in an office in town. Money had not been spared in setting up this hospital, it was plain to see.

When we visited the laundry in the basement of the male Chronic Building, the farthest one, I also saw the bakery where bread was made. Male patients worked in both these operations, under hired experienced supervisors. "There's a tailor shop where the men's outfits are made, and a shoe repair going full blast," Dawson told me. "And a Laboratory and Dispensary - as in the Female Chronic - an X-Ray department and Physiotherapy - they're in the Acute Building. All with experts in charge. You'll learn it all in time. I've been here over a year and I haven't been in some of the places I mentioned yet."

We did see the physiotherapy department the next day, as Mrs. Ridley was taken for hydrotherapy treatments. "It's immersion in warm water, and the tap is running all the time while the water drains out - very soothing for agitated patients," Dawson explained on the way over. "There's specially-equipped tubs on some of the wards in our building. I've seen women so disturbed that they've torn themselves out of the sheets they're wrapped in. Canvas sheets, I should say. Can you believe canvas being ripped apart? Well, I've seen it."

I was not looking forward to seeing anything of the sort and was glad that we didn't have any problem with Mrs. Ridley. I was interested in the prolonged sedative bath our patient was being given. She was wrapped in sheets and suspended in a canvas hammock in thermostatically-controlled running water. "When you hear about inhumane wet-sheet treatments," she said, "the patients have actually been in a soothing bath, but are so often experiencing delusions about torture that their stories are not factual at all."

One of the technicians proudly showed us their equipment. "We have tonic baths for stimulative muscle therapy, and we can give massage and exercises either alone or in combination with hydrotherapy," the physiotherapist explained. The tonic suite she was showing us was also equipped with the necessary apparatus for Light Therapy. There was a mercury quartz lamp for ultra-violet treatments, and infra-red lamps. "For muscle therapy, and the relief of pain. And there's a short-wave machine in the next room. Have you seen the chiropody room? There are mobile physio units that take treatments right to the wards, especially to the male and female infirmaries." We left Mrs. Ridley in the competent hands of the physiotherapists, to pick her up later. I realized that the newest methods and newest equipment were in use in the provincial mental hospital.

From all I heard from other nurses and from Fraser's constant complaining, I realized H2 was truly a 'good' ward as Gladwin had described it on my first morning. I was soon moving about without a thought of danger. The worst predicament in which I found myself was when one of my apron ends became caught in a door as it slammed shut behind me. I twisted around until I managed to get my key in the lock, and was able to laugh as I told Gladwin about it.

"You're lucky you were coming into an empty hall," my friend said soberly. "There's lots of patients would take advantage of you. You move too fast anyway." Gladwin, it's true, never hurried, but that was her nature. I was careful in doorways after that, but I was not able to curb my exuberance entirely.

Richmond spoke to me one day. "Nurses don't swing their keys around in a circle," she said. I detected a smile behind her serious manner. "And they don't whistle going down corridors, even if there are no patients to hear you. You like working here, don't you?"

I hadn't thought about it, but I realized the days were going very pleasantly. Richmond had one more admonition, given in her strictest voice. "And, Lehman, keep your key ring in your pocket, not outside your apron with the key tucked in your belt." I looked down, and sure enough, there was my key in my starched belt with the strap hanging untidily outside the slit in my apron. I hastily put it away.

I had been on ward H2 for several days, when the phone rang as I was coming out of the staff washroom through the office. Miss Coghlan was off and no one else was around so I picked up the receiver and said blithely, "H2. Lehman speaking."

To my surprise, Miss Hicks was on the line. "That's fine, Miss Lehman. You will do just fine. I want you to take a patient with a bucket of suds and a mop to wash the stairway by my office. Don't do it yourself." She spoke emphatically. "You know someone who will do it, don't you?" She gave me further instructions about locating the stairway and said she wanted it cleaned from top to bottom, then hung up.

I had not expected anything like this or I would have let the phone ring. I found Richmond and told her what I had been asked to do, then took a pleasant little woman called Bunny, one of the dayroom workers, to the utility room to get a mop. She said, "I'd rather just use a scrub brush and a cloth on a stairway, Miss Lehman. A mop would be awkward." We found Miss Hick's private stairway and started at the top to work down five floors.

That is, Bunny started to work. I spent a dreary hour standing by. If the Superintendent hadn't said so firmly that I was not to do it myself, I would have taken another bucket and shared the task. Why would she say I should not?

Then I remembered: The previous day Miss Coghlan had sent me to clean up an outside courtyard at the back of our ward. I had taken Bunny then, too, and enough mops and brooms so I could work with her. Had Miss Hicks seen me sweeping?

I would never know, but I accepted it all with good heart, and on my first day off reported my experiences cheerfully to my parents, much to their relief. When I returned to the Home on the early bus I bounded up the stairs to see what was going on in the dorm. I was actually glad to be back.

Some decisions made about the women patients were hard to understand. While Dawson and I were out on errands I saw male patients out without an attendant. "Ground privileges," Dawson said. "None for the women, though. I guess it would create problems. But couldn't they alternate days, or something? It makes me so mad!" Dawson was a vivacious little nurse, her curly hair bouncing with her lively movements as she shook her head crossly.

"Don't the women have any recreation besides a supervised walk once in a blue moon?" I asked.

"There are dances once a week in the winter months," Dawson said. "And concerts by the Red Cross. Now that summer is coming, there'll be outdoor concerts, bands playing on the lawns. But there always have to be nurses with the women when they're outside, so they don't get out very often." Neither did the nurses, I thought. And after a 12-hour day, mostly on our feet, we didn't care for much more than a short walk to get some fresh air.

Another probie had arrived in the dormitory - Renfrew, the self-confident girl I'd met while we were making out our applications. She had no more than a nod for me, hanging around Dunbar who wasn't really her type but who had gone to the same High School as Renfrew had. I was relieved when Renfrew was assigned to the other 'good' ward, F2, for her orientation.

Gladwin was going to be working on ward F3 for her regular assignment. The patients on F3 would be better than the ones on the top floor but not as good as those on the first floor.

"It could have been worse," Gladwin said. "The top floor wards won't see me for the next four months, at least. Maybe longer."

The next new girl to arrive was an enigma, and she was assigned to H2. It was my turn to help the newest probie learn the ward routine. Her name was Walford.

Walford was not only reserved, but she was totally unresponsive to any overtures of friendship. She picked up her bed linens the first night and I went over to help her make her bed. "Thanks, I can manage," she stated firmly, pushing in front of me to tuck in the sheet on my side. Repulsed, I retreated, and she was left alone to unpack and get ready for bed. Then Walford sat down in front of her mirror, painstakingly pinning her curls in place.

Her glossy black hair was combed straight back from her face to three rows of tight sausage curls from ear to ear at the back of her head. Walford was combing out each one, rolling it up again over her finger, and placing a bobby pin in it to hold it in place overnight. There must have been about two dozen small rolls to do.

Oliver watched silently for a few minutes. Then she put down her book and went to the new girl. "I'll put pins in for you, Walford. Don't your arms get tired holding them up?"

Oliver received the same rebuff I had - "I can manage, thank you." That was the last offer of help anyone made.

Walford was quick to pick up the ward routine, working with each nurse in turn. Richmond was puzzled. "I felt like I was giving a lecture. There was no response, and she didn't ask any questions. It's uncanny, talking to someone who doesn't even look you in the eye. When she was asked a question, her answer was as brief as possible." It wasn't shyness, as Walford was very self-possessed. "It's as if she has been badly hurt, and has built a wall between herself and other people," Oliver decided. We could always depend on Oliver for good advice. Now she outlined the course we would take with the new girl. "We'll just keep on being friendly. Everyone needs friends. She always answers though she never speaks first. I don't think we should ignore her. She's repressing her feelings, terribly, and probably afraid that if she starts talking she'll spill all her troubles. When the dam does burst - look out!"

Oliver was the philosopher in our little group. We called her our Corrections Officer for she reasoned out our behavior with incontrovertible logic which often had us squirming with sudden self-knowledge. She never relaxed her own overly-upright posture, but had such a pleasant way of speaking that we had to accept her remarks more as an expression of her own personality than as criticisms of ourselves.

Two more girls joined us in quick succession, Hammond and Ferrier. Hammond was tall and willowy, with straight fair hair pinned back behind her ears. She and Oliver became fast friends, forming quite a contrast in height, coloring, and posture. Hammond moved gracefully as she walked, while Oliver's shoulders were kept unrelentingly straight. They asked to be roommates when they moved out of the dormitory, and only once in the three years of their close relationship did we hear Hammond burst out, "I am so tired of everything I do or say being analyzed!" Oliver merely smiled, and the friendship continued as before.

Ferrier was a character who made her presence felt - and heard - immediately. Her sharp features wore an expression of incredulity after Miss Whitehorse had introduced her to the dormitory with her usual admonitions and complaints, and had fussed her way out again. We had all stood, as required by hospital rules, while the Home Supervisor was present, and Ferrier was the first to speak the minute Miss Whitehorse was gone.

"She's not for real, is she?" Ferrier was staring after the elderly nurse. "And that name! Guess it suits her at that. She's a nag."

"That's good. I like that." Dunbar was delighted. "Or Whitey Hee-Haw. Brays like a donkey!" The two girls looked at each other approvingly. And truly they were kindred spirits for Ferrier had no inhibitions. She stripped off her clothes except for her panties before she started to unpack, startling us by cradling her breasts - magnificent specimens indeed - in her hands as she crooned, "There, Dolly. There, Della. You don't like that awful brassiere any more than I do, do you? That feels better, doesn't it?" Complacently she turned to her unpacking.

I was fascinated by her outrageous behavior, designed to shock us, and intrigued by her flaunting of a figure which had none of the rounded softness of Dunbar's. I could see why she wanted to remove her bra, for the straps had cut into her shoulders cruelly. Otherwise Ferrier was as slim as a young boy, flat-hipped, with long legs that were very little larger above the knee than below.

Ferrier and Dunbar teamed up immediately. They were the only ones in the dorm who wore a garter belt. The rest of us, whatever our figure, pulled on an elastic girdle with garters attached to hold up our lisle stockings - nylons were not yet on the market, and the comforts of pantyhose were four decades in the future. Either way, garter belt or girdle, we all endured an expanse of bare flesh from the top of our stockings to the edge of our panties, for we would not wear the bloomers of our mothers' day.

The tube-like elastic girdles were a great improvement over the contraptions our mothers laced themselves into, at that. One-piece, from under the arms to below the hips, the old-time corsets were instruments of torture, we thought.

We were discussing Ferrier at the breakfast table, keeping a cautious eye out for her appearance. Dunbar was not present, nor Renfrew. Fraser had noted how Renfrew hovered around the other two, but did not disrobe so freely.

"Her figure isn't as good," sniffed Fraser. "If she was ten or fifteen pounds lighter, she'd have her clothes off too."

"That's probably true of most of us," Gladwin said, and Fraser had the grace to blush.

Oliver, whose upright posture even at the table always added weight to her pronouncements, stated, "Ferrier wants to draw attention to herself. Dunbar is just anxious to prove how sophisticated she is." That seemed to sum it up quite well.

We felt sorry for the next probie to arrive before she so much as opened her mouth to speak. Her pale skin was flushed crimson by the time she came into the dorm behind the expostulating Miss Whitehorse. Vanderhoof's fair hair was wound in thin braids around her head. She kept her head lowered as if afraid to face us, her whole appearance one of uncertainty and doubt. How well I remembered that feeling of apprehension, even dread, and I determined to give her all the help of which I was capable. This proved to be something I could do, for Walford was moved to a new ward before I was, and Vanderhoof came to H2 for her initial training while I was still there.

She was willing to learn and anxious to please, and a relief to all of us after dealing with her self-contained aloof predecessor.

Kelsey and Langley had moved out of the dormitory to a room on the second floor, and Gladwin and I, who had already put in a request to be roommates when our turn came, went down to see it. Most of the rooms were doubles, though the Charge Nurses had single rooms, as did a few of the graduates who had stayed on as staff members.

It was an attractive room, comfortably appointed. The door from the hall opened beside two clothes cupboards built out from the wall, with a washbasin fitted in neatly between them. Dark blue drapes on the double windows matched the blue patterned rug covering most of the hardwood floor. The beds were positioned opposite the cupboards, and large framed pictures hung on the walls. Blue bedspreads completed a carefully planned decorative scheme.

"We have to clean it ourselves," Kelsey told us. "The door is supposed to be locked when we're not here. It's much handier to the washrooms." We looked it over enviously.

"I can't wait to get a room of our own," Gladwin said on our way back to the dorm.

"Me too," I agreed. "Though I must say I've learned a lot there, about how different the girls are and about human nature in general. Just going to school with them wasn't nearly so revealing."

"A good choice of words, Lehman! How right you are!" She wound a friendly arm around my waist, and we knew we'd get along well.

While still in the dormitory we all found notices in our mailboxes informing us that we were to report, in full uniform, at eight o'clock the next night for a physical, on ward F2.

"Have you ever had a physical?" I asked. I hadn't, and didn't know what to expect.

"Nope. But my kid brother did, when he got a summer job with the CNR. He was only 14." She was giving little spurts of laughter, and my curiosity was aroused.

"Well, tell me about it," I said impatiently. "And what's so funny?" Gladwin was still gurgling to herself.

"OK, but for Pete's sake, don't tell it around. He's terribly embarrassed about it, and he'd be teased unmercifully if his friends got wind of it."

It was amusing, and I was laughing too when I heard it all. His mother had gone with the boy, knowing he had never been to a doctor in his healthy young life. Everything went well until he was handed a bottle and told to go into the bathroom and fill it, and she could see he was puzzled. However, he didn't ask any questions and she thought he'd be able to figure it out. She knew he hadn't when he stuck his head out of the bathroom door to ask, "Hot or cold?"

Poor kid! I wondered aloud, "What would a 14-year old boy be hired to do for the Canadian National Railway?"

"Just cleaning up in the roundhouse, I think," Gladwin answered. "He still works there in the summer, and we hope he'll be taken on steady when he's through school."

Our physical could have been worse, but was embarrassing enough for most of us as we had to strip to the waist. Miss Marlatt gave us a towel to put over our shoulders while we waited to be summoned for our turn. We were in the visitors' room on F2 which was on the same floor as H2 but on the opposite side. The floor plan was a reversal of H2, which felt rather strange. Miss Marlatt took us in to the doctor in turn, Fraser first. Dunbar and Ferrier started teasing Vanderhoof.

"Look! She's blushing, all the way down to her waist! Keep a good hold on that towel, Vanderhoof." Dunbar's smile was diabolic. "The doctor doesn't have to see you. Let him feel up underneath the towel."

Ferrier joined in with, "Yeah, and watch out for other 'feels' like under your skirt. Say, you know why women have always worn skirts, since cave man days, don't you?" Her eyes were sparkling with mischief. "Who do you suppose made the rules? The men, of course! So's the women would be readily available..."

Oliver intervened severely. "Cut it out, you two. That's not funny." Miss Marlatt returned just then and took Dunbar next, and Fraser got dressed again. "I'll wait for you, Gladwin." She noticed Vanderhoof's scarlet face and said kindly, "Hey, there's nothing to worry about." We all plied Fraser with questions and Ferrier was forgotten.

When my turn came to be taken across the hall by Miss Marlatt, I was met by Miss Hicks who sat me on a stool facing Dr. Campbell, who was also seated. "This is Miss Lehman," she said, and whisked off the towel. She remained behind me, keeping her hand on my shoulder for a moment in a reassuring gesture. With her in attendance, the examination by stethoscope was not so bad. Then I had to turn my back and cough as directed while he thumped the lung area. Miss Hicks returned my towel and I answered questions about childhood diseases. Dr. Campbell was young, very good-looking, with fair hair carefully parted and waved. His final question, "Do you have any trouble with your periods?" being answered in the negative, I was free to go.

Gladwin and Fraser were waiting to walk back with me, already in possession of the bottle. Miss Marlatt was handing them out with instructions to leave them at the Information desk in the morning. "Be sure to put your name on the label," she cautioned.

We had a discussion of childhood diseases on the way back to the Home. Oliver and Hammond were with us. We'd all had chickenpox and measles - two kinds, Oliver said grimly. "The red measles were the worst."

"I was in quarantine for measles for six weeks," Gladwin said. "The first three while my brother had it, then three more when I got it just as we were ready to go back to school."

"Did you have to line up for small-pox vaccinations at school?" I asked. "I never knew anyone to get small-pox, but I had a cousin die from diphtheria. The doctor had to come five miles on bad roads - my uncle had to go and get him because we didn't have telephones in the country at that time. So the poor kid choked to death before the doctor got there."

Back in the dormitory there was much hilarity about the urine specimens. "How are we supposed to fill these dinky bottles?" Ferrier wanted to know. "It looks like a pretty messy business to me. Say, does anyone know where there's a bedpan?"

"I do," Renfrew contributed eagerly. "I saw one in the supply room when I picked up my uniform."

"Wouldn't it be a lark to all pee in the same pan and fill our bottles from that?" Ferrier chortled. "D'you think they'd notice?"

Judging from the giggles in the morning as we placed our bottles on the Information desk, the three conspirators did just that, but there were no repercussions. They were quite disappointed. "They probably wanted to find out if anyone was pregnant," Ferrier grumbled.

Before I left ward H2, I discovered what "Help on J!" entailed. Dawson and I were returning to the ward from an errand when Miss Coghlan met us in the rotunda. "Help on J!" she said to Dawson. "And you go too, Lehman."

Dawson turned to the stairway off the rotunda and with me pounding at her heels we ran up two flights of stairs. We crossed ward H4 rotunda and ran down the hall to the door that would have led into the dining room on our floor. Here we were in ward J, and all I could see were closed doors on either side of a long corridor. This was a ward of side-rooms, forty single cells bare of furniture, for violent patients.

The noise of a wild altercation drew us, on the run, to the room where help was needed, to a scene I could never have imagined. Five or six nurses were trying to quell a kicking, cursing, furious woman. They had her on the floor, but she wasn't subdued. She twisted and turned and bucked them off with unbelievable strength. Dawson threw herself on to one leg and I added my weight to the other, and felt myself lifted up in spite of the fact there were two of us on that limb. The Charge nurse was standing by with a hypodermic, waiting for a chance to plunge it in.

Two more nurses ran in and the Charge saw her opportunity. "Try to turn her over," she said, "and bare her bottom." Every one of us was needed to control this rampaging creature, but somehow we turned her over and the needle was driven into her buttock.

Dawson tugged at my arm and we slipped out one by one before the woman could get up and charge at the door which was closed in her face. There was a handle on the outside that turned a lock, then a key completed the safeguard against her delirious madness.

"That's maniacal strength," Dawson remarked, straightening her cap and smoothing her apron as we walked back to H2. "You have no idea how strong a person can get until you see one in a blind frenzy like that. She'll drop off to sleep now, and may need more shots for a few days until her violent phase is over. Then she won't remember much of this except as part of the persecution she's imagining. I'll never understand what gets into them."

Back on the ward, I looked at my fellow nurses with a new respect and a strong sense of fellowship. Together we were dealing with the problems of the mentally ill. We really needed each other.

At the end of the month, after two weeks on H2, there were three major events in my life. I received my first pay envelope, with all of $16 in it, the first money I ever had to spend on myself. At a time when a good wool suit cost $12, when merchants were going out of business for lack of customers, when a working man counted himself lucky to make a dollar for a ten-hour day, this was good money. My first pay seemed like a fortune.

Next, Gladwin and I were moved to a room of our own, on the first floor. The very first night Gladwin surprised me by saying, "Let's sleep together! I don't see why not." I agreed, and we spent a very uncomfortable night in one single bed, much too crowded but determined to countermand Miss Whitehorse's, to us, inexplicable orders. That over, we settled into our room with pleasure. Gladwin was a sensible person and there was a keen sense of humor under her sober exterior. We had three happy years together.

The third major event was a new assignment. For the next several months I would be on ward F4, the ward Fraser hated so much.

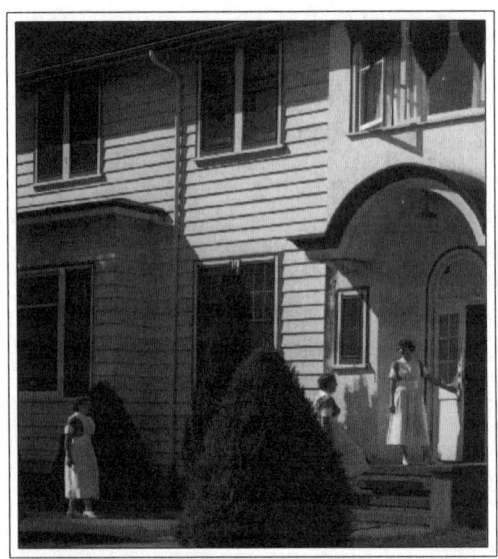

Student nurses at the Nurses' Home

CHAPTER FIVE

The top floor wards, H4, J and F4, were known to be the worst to work on. On H4 and J the patients were prone to violence. On F4 it was disease. Some of the women were in the last stages of syphilis, marked by deterioration mentally and physically. And an even larger number had tuberculosis as well as the dementia praecox symptoms that led to hospitalization at Essondale. Eventually ward F4 was turned into a TB ward and the nurses wore protective nose-and-mouth masks on duty. But we ran the risks unknowingly. My chest X-Rays today show scarred lungs and TB skin tests are still wildly positive, but apparently my system overcame the disease successfully.

Fraser was still on F4, though her plans to marry were definite and she would be leaving in two weeks. Keith, the Charge Nurse, was probably in her 40s. Her homely appearance was mitigated by complete dedication to her work. Her concern for patients and staff alike was unremitting. As I came into the living room before roll-call that morning she had said, "Welcome to F4, Lehman." Her voice, with a Scots accent, was cheery yet brisk and business-like. She had a gift for commanding love and respect, and I became her ardent admirer.

Fraser initiated me into the morning routine, which consisted of rounding up stragglers from the dormitory and making them presentable for the day. So many of these dishevelled and unkempt women needed assistance in dressing and personal care that the night staff of only two nurses could not possibly handle them all. A sorrier lot than these couldn't be envisioned. The majority had no interest in their appearance or their surroundings. Many stared vacantly into space, some revealed their inner disturbances by their moving lips or facial grimaces. The better patients were already in the dayroom and my first impressions were of the wretched remainder.

Breakfast was a revelation in gross behavior. The dining room for wards F4 and H4 was halfway between them, over the office area two floors below. "Ward J get their meals on trays," Fraser explained. "They can't be let out of their cells in their violent state."

When I came into the patients' breakfast, leading two women who would not move on their own, a noisy, slovenly mob greeted my eyes and ears. The first to arrive gobbled their food in order to grab from the plates around them, and the nurses from both wards were kept busy preventing, or trying to settle, the quarrels that arose. One mannerism of many of the women at their meals disgusted me, and I never saw it without revulsion. This was a compulsion on the part of some women to mix everything together into a revolting mess before starting to eat. This was shovelled into a mouth that was lowered almost to the plate to receive it. Huge mouthfuls were swallowed without chewing, in gulp after greedy gulp.

My task was to feed catatonic patients. Fraser was also spooning food into passive women, and she explained their condition. "When they're completely catatonic they are like statues. They can stand or sit for hours without moving, and they don't even seem to see although their eyes are open. So they have to be washed, dressed, and fed. I was told they can get into a state of excitement, but I haven't seen any such thing while I've been here." Fraser was very gentle with the women. It was apparent that the more aggressive patients were across the hallway on ward H4, but they were not quite as messy as ours.

Once back on the ward, I was introduced to the toilet routine after meals. There were six stalls and the lack of doors on them was of great help on this ward, for almost all the women had to be herded through. Fraser was putting the most passive ones on and off the toilets, and I saw that she painstakingly wiped a few bottoms, as she had told us. When that task fell to me, I found that handing out toilet paper and then ignoring the women produced an automatic response to this personal need.

A cranky-looking older nurse with obviously dyed hair - the roots were gray and the color too black - was stationed inside the washroom door, moving the women along the line. "Keep them coming, Lehman!" she glared at me, her face set in a crabbed, churlish expression. "We don't want to be here all day."

On my very first morning I was 'keeping them coming' and one bumped into Skyler, inside the door. She gave me a look of pure venom, and snapped, "Look where you're pushing, Lehman! You're just as careless as the others. You'd better watch out, or I'll show you what pushing is!" Thoroughly chastened, I escaped to the office as soon as the last woman was through.

There I was met by Miss Keith. "You can go to breakfast, Lehman," she told me. "Hardy is waiting for you; she'll show you where to get antiseptic soap to scrub your hands. And don't let Skyler bother you," she said to my surprise. I was to discover that Keith knew everything that happened on her ward. Her eyes twinkled as she added, "When you're 45 and going through the change-of-life you could be cranky too." She laughed with me.

Hardy, unapologetically plump, was as comfortable as an old grandmother. She had protruding eyes, a wide, slack mouth, and a habit of looking sideways at you after she spoke as if uncertain of your reaction. She too, had heard Skyler's dressing-down and advised me to pay no attention. "We all get heck from Skyler," she shrugged. "Forget it. She's always crabby." I warmed to Hardy's friendship.

The dayroom assignment on F4 was monotonous for most of the women were sunk into apathy by their physical deterioration. Even the women who did the ward work were of a phlegmatic nature, tackling the most disagreeable tasks without seeming to mind.

Keith came up to me with a pair of heavy ward stockings in her hand. "See that everyone is presentable for rounds," she said in her pleasant Scottish burr. "Use a ward comb - their heads are perfectly clean; they get showered and shampooed every few days. And put these stockings on Mrs. Brown." She pointed out a bare-legged women whose head hung down dejectedly, her dress on inside-out. "Let's get that dress on the right way, Mrs. Brown," Keith pulled her to her feet, and I helped her right the dress.

Keith's willingness to work along side her nurses in pursuing her relentless goal of scrupulous patient care endeared her to the staff.

I would have done anything she asked, for I knew she would do it too.

After pulling the stockings over the open sores on Mrs. Brown's legs, I went directly for the antiseptic soap and scrubbed my hands. In spite of our precautions we developed scabies on ward F4, which we treated with straight Lysol as soon as we saw it. We then had to resort to creams and lotions to soothe the skin, but the hated scabies was conquered. Until the next time.

It was on F4 that I met Marshall, who became my mentor, friend, and guide to leisure activities, making me aware of many healthy ways to counteract our long hours indoors. Marshall was starting her third year and was a most efficient nurse, a hard worker who often became impatient of accepted routines and devised short-cuts to everyone's advantage. Her usual purposeful expression had produced a permanent frown which remained on her forehead even when she was cheerfully smiling. On this first morning she was in the dayroom smartening up the patients for the doctor's round.

"There, they look presentable, Lehman," she told me briskly. "Now we just fade into the background and hope the doctor comes soon. Mrs. Brown will have her stockings off before too long. Keep an eye on her." She stayed with me, filling in details about various women who needed attention.

To my surprise Keith was not with Dr. Ryan and his usual escort of Miss Hicks and Miss Marlatt. A dainty nurse in an all-white uniform, as immaculate as the other two, accompanied them. "Who is that?" I asked Marshall, who was standing beside me.

"Miss Courtenay, our Supervisor," Marshall explained with a grin. "I don't wonder you haven't seen her. She's a registered nurse. There's one on every ward except F2 and H2. They take a post-graduate course in psych nursing here and some were picked for Supervisors. They aren't here before breakfast, and they take a two-hour lunch, and go off early. Pretty soft job, I'd say. You don't see them at roll-call because they don't live in the Nurses' Home. They have rooms in this building, right above the office area. Yeah, that's below the F4-H4 dining room, with all its noise and commotion. They complain about the elevator, too, the ones whose rooms are close to it. I don't feel sorry for them! Miss Courtenay's nice, though.

They all are, actually. Why shouldn't they be? It's a soft job."

Three hectic meal-times followed by the toilet parade, an afternoon spent on spit-and-polish wherever Keith deemed it necessary, laundry and drugs pick-up and other errands, linen room folding and storing, showers from supper-time until the night staff came on - all this made a long and tiring day. Keith was indefatigable, doing as much as any of her staff, and her standards were high. By the end of the day my feet were aching, and she noticed it.

"Come with me, Lehman," she said, leading me to the dispensary down the corridor. "Here, I've poured a formaldehyde solution into this bottle. This cork will fit it; there you are. Soak your feet for half an hour or longer in warm water, and put a dollop of this in it. Not too much, mind you. It's strong stuff. That will toughen up your feet."

I found a basin in the storeroom at the Nurses' home and had just eased my sore feet into the soothing warmth when a senior nurse looked into the open door of our room. Gladwin had gone down to the kitchen to make tea for us and I was alone.

"Hi! Your name's Lehman, isn't it? I'm Sullivan, on H4. I've seen you across the patients' dining room. How would you like to come out dancing tonight? One of the fellows needs a partner." She smiled encouragingly.

I was tempted, and flattered to be asked. Sullivan was an exceptionally pretty girl with tight red curls and a milky complexion lightly sprinkled with freckles. She added, "You know how to get in by the fire-escape, don't you? I landed on your bed one night. We probably won't come back together."

Oh, yes, Sullivan! The girl who had frightened the wits out of me my first night in the dormitory. "It's perfectly safe, you know," she added, seeing my hesitation. "Old Whitey is busy with her midnight meal, then she nods off. She'd never go up those stairs."

My love of dancing had almost won out over my sore feet, but the idea of sneaking in late decided me. "Gee, thanks, Sullivan. I'd sure love to go, but my feet are killing me and I just couldn't tonight. I hope you'll ask me another time." Sullivan went off in search of another lucky girl and I felt like a real wet blanket. Maybe I'd been foolish to turn her down.

Almost on Sullivan's heels, Keith popped into my room. She was still in her uniform. "Lehman, was Sullivan asking you to go out with her? She was? You didn't say you would, did you? She's bad news! In more ways than one! First of all she'd take you to a beer parlor, and you're not 21. Are you? And ten-to-one you'd be late getting back, and that's dynamite for your chances of passing your probation here, and being kept on. And there's something else." She paused, as if deciding how to say it.

"I don't think I've mentioned this yet, Lehman. I always tell the new girls on my ward to be careful of toilet seats! There are nearly 100 girls in this Home, and a few aren't the kind I'd want to see you become. They could have venereal disease. You know what that is, don't you? We all use the same washrooms and toilets. Just be careful, I'm telling you. And stay away from Sullivan and her crowd!" Keith was gone, before I could mumble a thank you.

What a close call I'd had! Keith's advice led to a life-long phobia on my part about toilet seats. If I had to sit on the ones in the Home I piled layers of toilet paper on them. But I couldn't tell even my roommate about the warning. It seemed shameful to be working with girls who might have venereal disease, though my common sense told me very few even had boyfriends in those days when money was scarce. So how could they be diseased?

Two weeks sped by, and Fraser left. "I'll be in touch with you," she said to Gladwin and me. "I want you to come and visit, and stay overnight when you can. Stan works four hours a day, and I'll be lonely."

"Still complaining!" Oliver remarked when we told the others at the breakfast table. "Fraser won't be any happier married than she was here." But I had seen a new side of Fraser on the ward, and I wondered. Time would tell.

With Fraser gone, timid little Vanderhoof was assigned to our ward, and I was given Fraser's former task of taking meal trays to the side-room patients in the dormitory. The top floor wards, apart from ward J which was all side-rooms, each had six single rooms with the same peep-hole arrangement as on J. This was a small round window with wire-reinforced glass. The door locked from outside by turning the handle, with a key lock as a final measure of safety. These were used on a short-term basis for our own patients when they became obstreperous.

Each side-room had a regular-sized outer window with a section that opened out for ventilation. There was no furniture for the patient to use against us or to hurt herself with while in a frenzy. A blanket was provided at night and meals were brought on trays.

The task of giving out trays and picking them up when empty appeared much easier and more pleasant than the dining room hassle, and I was pleased. I did not anticipate any problem as the dormitory was quiet. The women were probably sedated. I unlocked each door, slid the tray onto the floor and carefully locked the door again.

I wheeled the trolley back to the first cell and started collecting trays when a glance through the peep-hole showed the woman had eaten. Five trays were picked up without trouble and only one remained. There, Mrs. Abbott was crouched against the wall, a picture of despair with her head buried in her arms which rested on her drawn-up knees. She was quite a young woman, dishevelled now but lithe and attractive.

I unlocked the door and saw that the tray was under the window. Unsuspecting, I walked over and bent down to pick it up. I was straightening up when I heard the door slam shut and the handle turn, and I despairingly realized that I had been outwitted by the young woman. She was out in the corridor, and I was locked in a side-room.

I ran to unlock the door and found that the key-hole did not extend to the inside, which was perfectly smooth. My precious key was of no use at all.

Helplessly I peered out of the peep-hole and witnessed my patient smashing the glass on the dormitory window across the corridor. She broke out a jagged piece of glass and proceeded to draw it over one wrist, then the other.

I ran to the window to call for help, but the dormitory was at the back of the building and there was no one in sight. Even as my mind registered that fact, I realized that hollering from windows was disregarded by passers-by, and even in my predicament I could see the improbability of the message, "I'm a nurse. I've been locked in!" being taken seriously. My humiliation was indescribable.

I ran back to the door and incredibly it was opened by Mrs. Abbott, who turned the handle to show me her bleeding wrists. "Now what are you going to do?" she asked. I wasted no time in leaving that room, grabbing her arms tightly above the cuts to contain the bleeding as much as possible. With her beside me, my right hand grasping her right arm and my left hand on her left arm, I rushed her to the ward office.

There was no one there, no one in the dayrooms. The ward was at dinner, all patients and all nurses. I went down the corridor and to my great relief the surgery door was open, and Miss Courtenay was there. She took charge bandaging the cuts, which were not deep.

After hearing my story she said kindly, "I don't suppose I have to tell you now not to go inside a side-room to remove a tray. Make the patient leave it beside the door." Keith had returned by this time and she added, "I'm sure Lehman has learned a lesson," Both of them were smiling. I knew I had been let off easily and I was fortunate in having Miss Courtenay and Keith on the ward. They didn't let my secret out though it probably was reported to Miss Hicks and Dr. Ryan, but it wasn't on the day report and I was never teased by the other nurses. I certainly kept it quiet, telling only Gladwin, and she told no one. A true pal.

Keith did talk to me about the vigilance needed on the wards. "You can't trust any of them," she said. "I know that's hard to believe with some of the workers who would do anything for us, but they do go 'off' and it's not always easy to read the signs ahead of time." We had returned Mrs. Abbott to the side-room, sedated and with a blanket to sleep in.

"Why would Mrs. Abbott, a young attractive woman, want to commit suicide?" I asked.

"She didn't really want to die," answered Keith, "or she would have cut deeper. Miss Courtenay said the blood wasn't spurting, just trickling. She's done this before, you know. She does it to attract attention. She's post-partum depressive and should get better, though it has taken longer with each baby. She's had four, and she's only in her early 20s. I'll have to phone maintenance to replace the glass." She hurried off, and I returned to my tasks.

Mrs. Abbott was back in the dayroom several days later and I had an opportunity to sit with her. "I'm glad you're feeling better, Mrs. Abbott. Are you looking forward to going home soon?"

"No! No! Not back home! That's where the torture room is!" her face twisted into a knot of fear. "It's dark, they use knives, and red-hot pokers. You don't know how cruel they can be!" She moaned softly. I realized she was not only depressed, she was delusional. No, she was not better yet.

My second pay envelope contained $33, a full month's pay. I waltzed down the hallway of the Nurses' Home, whistling happily as I thought of all I could buy. A white sweater, for cool rainy days. White stockings, which cost nearly $2 a pair, and developed runs which had to be mended. Put a few dollars away for the dentist - I was paying my own bills now.

Skyler was coming toward me and I stopped whistling and side-stepped to go by, but she stepped in front of me. "I say, Lehman, could you lend me ten dollars? My sister in Penticton is sick and I need bus fare to go and see her."

Skyler was actually begging me for a favor! Would she be easier on me on the ward if I loaned her the money?

"Could you let me have it now? I'm off the next two days and I want to catch the next bus to town to get the midnight bus to the Okanagan. I'll have it back to you next week."

How could I refuse? There went my hopes for a sweater. "OK, Skyler. I'll go and get it now." "Bring it to my room, will you? I have to pack," and she turned into her room a few doors from mine.

Miss Keith appeared and followed me into my room. "Lehman, did I see Skyler talking to you? Was she asking for a loan? How much? Ten dollars! Listen, don't give her a red cent. She'll never pay you back."

I started to explain. "Her sister is sick..."

"Sister! Don't you believe it! Skyler wouldn't help her ailing mother! She has a different story every time."

"But what will I do?" I wailed. "She's waiting for me. I said I'd take it to her room." What had I gotten into?

"Just march in there and tell her you can't spare it! Why should she need money today? She got paid too, didn't she? And she makes more than you do."

Feeling like a fool I approached Skyler's room. Her door was open. She had seen Keith go into my room and she was furious. "Keith got hold of you, didn't she! Well, you can go to hell, both of you! I don't care," and she slammed her door in my face.

What a relief! I silently thanked Keith and berated myself for my gullibility. Skyler couldn't be worse than she already was on the ward, anyway. And I could get my sweater.

Vanderhoof had been on the ward for about six weeks and she was still not comfortable with the patients. She stayed close to me or any other nurse whenever possible, and cast fearful looks over her shoulder. I had forgotten my fear of being attacked from behind but Vanderhoof's behavior reminded me of my first day when I backed up against the wall. Keith was patiently trying to help her, giving her work in the dormitories rather than the dayrooms and sending her on errands off the ward, but inevitably Vanderhoof had to be with the patients much of the time. And she was scared.

One day we were in the dayroom and Vanderhoof confided to me, "I've got an awful rash on the fronts of my legs. Look, you can see the bumps under my stockings. The itch is driving me crazy!" She didn't look well, feverish and strained.

I was about to suggest she show the rash to Miss Courtenay when, true to her usual percipience, Keith came to us and said, "Come into the office, Vanderhoof. I want to look at the rash on your legs." Vanderhoof did not reappear on the ward that day and when I asked Keith, she said, "She's in bed in the Nurses' Home. Why don't you go and see her tonight?"

Her flushed face crimson against the pillow, Vanderhoof told me what had happened. Keith had sent her to Miss Hicks, who told her to go right over to the Home and go to bed. "And stay there," she said. "You can get up to the bathroom, and that's all. Your meals will be brought to you. I'll be over with Dr. Campbell to look at that rash."

"And what did Dr. Campbell say?" I asked, wondering if it was something contagious. Evidently not, for she could have visitors.

"He didn't say much, just that it's erythema nodosum. Miss Hicks wrote it down for me, after he left. She stayed to explain about it. She said I'd be off work for six months, and rest in bed the first two. And she asked if my parents could take me home. There is no nurses' infirmary here."

Vanderhoof had talked long enough and I left her to get her rest, as prescribed. She would be going home the next day.

On the ward the next day Marshall knew all about erythema nodosum. "I had it when I started, after a couple of months," she said. "Its cause is unknown, but there's a theory, my doctor told me, that it's a form of rheumatic fever, which is most often contracted by young nurses who have never been in contact with TB. The theory is that it's caused by an overdose of tuberculosis germs and it comes out in the rash that Vanderhoof had. And boy! Is it itchy! I had some rash on my arms too!"

"How long were you off?" I asked Marshall.

"Just over three months," was the surprising answer. "Miss Hicks phoned me and said she couldn't hold my job for me unless I got back before lectures started. When you think about it, it would mean missing a year of your training if you couldn't start lectures in September with the rest of your class. So I came back, and I've been fine. Awfully tired the first while, but that worked off."

"Do you think you had TB?" I asked.

Marshall's frown deepened. "All I know is that I had to have a chest X-Ray every three months the first year, and every six months now, for I don't know how long. No spots on my lungs. But you should see the reaction I get to the skin test. It's this wide," and she measured a couple of inches on her arm. "So I have been in contact with TB - haven't we all?" She laughed dryly. "Maybe I've developed an immunity. I'd like to think so."

It was a comfort to get an encouraging report on something that sounded so frightening. But we never saw Vanderhoof again. She did not return to work as a psychiatric nurse.

CHAPTER SIX

At the end of summer our probationary period was over and we were issued our wide bibs and caps. There was no capping ceremony, as in general hospital nursing. The new items were placed in our laundry compartments in the O.T., and Langley was the first to get hers after work. She had her clean laundry bag packed when I arrived.

"Surprise!" she sang out. "No more probie bibs! And CAPS!"

Gladwin and I were pinning clean collars and cuffs on to our clean uniform dresses that night, in our room. "I sure like these wide bibs," Gladwin said. "Those little square bibs are like baby bibs, I always thought. And I'm looking forward to wearing the cap."

"Yeah, but I never expected we'd have to sew our caps into shape," said Renfrew, looking at the flat semi-circular starched object in her hand. She had come to our room to borrow a needle and thread and stayed to do the sewing. "How many pleats are we supposed to put into them?"

"I've been looking at how the caps are pleated." Oliver spoke in her precise way. Hammond was away on days off and her roommate had come to spend the evening with us. She continued, "Have you noticed Salmon, the tall blond with her hair done into two buns, one over each ear?" After months of roll calls, we knew the names of all nurses in the Home.

"Well, she makes the tiniest pleats in her caps," said Oliver. "No one else I've seen makes them that small."

"Not for me," stated Renfrew emphatically. "I've got enough chores already, polishing white shoes and washing white stockings every night..."

"Just be thankful you don't have to wear black, like you would if you were training in a general hospital," broke in Gladwin. "They look so blah. I think we're lucky to have white. And I don't think it matters how many pleats you put in your cap, so long as it's gathered into shape. The caps all look different from the back."

"But I'll bet Miss Hicks notices," put in Oliver. "If you have only four or five big pleats she'll know you do them in a terrible hurry, not caring how it looks. I'm making mine small pleats, but not Salmon's tiny ones. I think they look neater when they're small. We only have to sew them in once a week anyway, when we get our clean laundry. A cap won't get mussed like our uniforms do."

We all looked at Gladwin in surprise when she started to laugh. "Lehman, tell them about your clean laundry this week," she sputtered.

"Ugh!" I shuddered. "It wasn't funny when I put my laundry bag down and a mouse jumped out. Right there by your feet, Renfrew," I added when I saw her look around fearfully. She drew her feet up onto the bed, and asked quickly, "Is it still here?" Her eyes were darting here and there.

"Relax, Renfrew. Do you think we're making a pet out of a mouse? Have a heart, Lehman, and tell her what happened."

"Well, I wanted to jump up on the bed, too, but I knew I had to get rid of that mouse, and luckily it darted out the door and ran down the hall, with me after it. I'd grabbed a shoe to throw at it. I saw it go into one of the rooms, and when I saw whose room, I got back here quick, and shut the door."

"Whose room?" asked Renfrew. "I didn't think you'd do anything like that, Lehman."

"Oh yes, I would and I did. Skyler's room, that's who."

"Poor mouse," murmured Oliver, and we all laughed.

"I guess you've all discovered how handy our laundry bags are for bringing over sanitary pads," said Renfrew, who had finished her cap and was applying some of my nail polish.

"You're taking sanitary pads from ward supplies?" asked Gladwin. "Aren't you afraid of getting caught?"

"Who's to catch me? I'm not the only one; everybody does it. It's one thing less to buy from our $37 a month." We had received a raise in wages along with our caps. "Say, did you know we'll get five dollars a month more on night duty?" Renfrew went on. "No one likes nights but the extra money helps."

Gladwin was still doubtful about taking pads off the wards. "I've never seen anyone swiping them. I don't believe everyone does."

"Sure they do," said Renfrew impatiently. "You don't see them because they slip them into their laundry bags, or bring them over under their capes on rainy days. You can get a lot of things under your cape. I'll bet some of the girls who leave to get married take blankets and towels too. New ones." She held up one hand to inspect her nails.

Oliver had been looking thoughtful, and her question showed she'd gone off into another line of thought. "How old were you when you started to menstruate?" she asked.

"Fourteen." "Twelve." The answers came together. Gladwin added, "And I didn't have a period the first three months I was here. Because working here was such a change, the doctor said." I was surprised; she hadn't said a word to me.

Oliver wouldn't be sidetracked. "I was ten," she confided. "Just about four months after my tenth birthday. I didn't even know what was happening. I was sleeping over at a neighbor's like I did sometimes when my parents were going out. I always slept with their household helper, Kitty. She had come from Scotland when she was about 16 or 17 years old, and she had the prettiest hair - auburn, with tight curls all over her head. She hated it, wanted waves if you can imagine." We had never heard Oliver talk this much; it seemed to be a release for her and no one interrupted.

"Anyway, in the morning the two kids came in and climbed all over us, a little girl and a little boy. All at once Kitty shooed them out to get dressed, and it was then I noticed big reddish-brown spots all over the sheet on my side of the bed. Dumb me, I asked, 'What's that?' 'Don't you know?' asked Kitty. 'Never mind, I'll walk home with you after breakfast. You said last night your tummy was sore.'" She was stripping the sheets off the bed.

"I guess Kitty had told her employer what was happening because Mrs. Bradner excused us from doing the dishes and Kitty came home with me. I couldn't hear what she was saying to my mother but I heard Mother say, 'I'm so sorry. I'll wash the sheets for you.

She's only ten years old!' 'Oh, no thank you,' Kitty said cheerfully. 'Mrs. Bradner won't mind; she said so. I'm the one who does the washing; I'll look after them.'"

Oliver's voice had been dry as she was talking but now the strain of what she was remembering showed as her voice cracked. "You won't believe the next part. After Kitty left, my mother was cross. 'You can expect this every month for the rest of your life. Kitty said you had a sore stomach so you'll likely get cramps every month too.' She handed me a folded cloth and pins. 'Pin that to your undershirt front and back.' That was all the sympathy or explanation I got."

"Weren't those cloth pads awful?" said Renfrew. We nodded. Our generation had been introduced to Kotex only a few years previously and most of us had been started with folded strips of old sheets or underwear which were bulky, uncomfortable, and probably very smelly. We had nothing to change into during a long school day.

"It was no fun washing out those cloths either," I added. "Ugh, I can still see the bloody water we had to plunge our hands into to wring the darn things out. Then they went into the copper boiler on the stove." We used wood stoves in the 30s.

"And wasn't it embarrassing to have to spread them out on the grass or hang them on bushes to dry," contributed Gladwin. "Everybody knew what they were."

"And once in awhile a girl would have a spot on the back of her skirt," I remembered. "My Grade 8 teacher had a spot on her dress one day. We saw it when she was writing on the blackboard."

"Didn't you tell her?" asked Oliver, her voice back to normal.

"Well, you know how embarrassed we were about it all. Three of us went to her together at recess, and she washed it out somehow. I don't know how because we had a pail of water for drinking, and outside toilets. Wasn't it awful?"

Renfrew had evidently given some thought to the problem of sanitary pads, or her idea was one that had been tossed about in High School. "You know, I'm as happy as you are that we don't have to wash the rags out but they could do better than that. Something like a little cup, a lot less messy than pads."

Gladwin snorted. "How about that? You're out on a date and you say, 'Excuse me, I have to go and empty my cup.'" Oliver was laughing too as she and Renfrew went out.

"I've never seen Oliver unbend so much," I remarked after they left. "She needed to get that off her chest."

"Learning about monthly periods is no fun for anyone," Gladwin said bleakly, as we gathered up soap and towels to go for a bath.

Before long we were in our beds with the lights out, a time for low-key conversation and exchange of confidences. Lectures would be starting the next evening. "Eight o'clock doesn't give us much time in the Home after work. We'll have to wear a uniform to lectures too, won't we?" I mused.

Gladwin sounded gloomy. "Have you thought about what it will mean on our days off?" she asked. "It will hardly be worth going home except on weekends, and you know very well we're lucky to get one weekend a month, and not always that."

"A couple more hours after work will make a long day," I acknowledged. I knew Gladwin was not as keen on lectures as I was. "But won't we be going on nights sometime this winter? Then we'll have lectures in our work hours."

"Yeah, but you don't get three meal-times on nights," retorted Gladwin. "So you have to go over for supper before work, and have your breakfast after you get off in the morning, and on days you get those meals in duty hours. And nights off will be worse for getting home. We have to sleep in the daytime so what's the use of going home when we have to be back for lectures five days of the week."

"It will sure cut into dating time," I thought aloud. I wasn't dating seriously, going to the movies or to an occasional dance with a shy young man who lived near my parents. He didn't have a car so I saw him only when I went home. I knew Gladwin was going with Don, a former schoolmate, and she seemed smitten. Gladwin was four years older than I.

"Darned lectures," groaned Gladwin. "Let's go to sleep." The room became quiet.

Lectures certainly did make a difference in our lives, but in spite of the curtailment of our time off, I found them fascinating and demanding. The lecture room was on the attic floor of the Female Chronic building, in the opposite wing to Occupational Therapy. Though I hadn't been to university, I imagined it was a typical lecture room, equipped with rows of chairs having one substantial arm rest for taking notes. Miss Hicks and Miss Marlatt attended all lectures, sitting quietly in the back row. Miss Marlatt marked our attendance in the Register during the lectures. It was all quite different from High School.

Dr. A.M.Gee, dark and compact, rather taciturn, lectured dryly on Psychology and Psychiatry, but this was so closely related to our work that it could not be dull. We never saw Dr. Gee except at lectures, as his work had to do with patients in the other two buildings. Now we could toss around terms like dementia praecox and schizophrenia, which had narrow meanings in the 30s. We saw signs of manic-depressive behaviour in one another, and dreaded old age because we saw so much senility with the custodial care in an institution for the mentally ill. We were, in turn, paranoid, hysterical, confused, disoriented, compensating, unstable, hyperactive, agitated, compulsive, and generally neurotic. Surely mental illness is a matter of degree. Ah, yes, we were told the criterion for admission is a breakdown of social skills, often judged by inherent danger to society caused by the aberration.

"The boundary line between the sane and the insane is too indistinct," I muttered one evening when Hammond was copying some psychiatry notes in our room. "How is it that we see a lot of this behaviour outside as well as in the wards?"

Gladwin picked up on my observation. "You must know the character in town who always wears a man's suit coat with a straight skirt of the same material." I nodded. "And she has a man's haircut, and her shoes are men's shoes. Everyone knows Miss Martin. She's a successful insurance agent. We have a hermaphrodite on ward F3 and she's treacherous; she'd as soon punch you as not. She has the powerful upper body and long arms of a man. The rest of her is a woman. I wonder about Miss Martin."

"I suppose being that way makes her hostile," said Hammond. "I know a strange man who could be a patient. He talks to himself. And he has such grandiose delusions. You know that big stone house on Kingsway, with the stone fence around the whole block, and the beautiful grounds? Well, he says he built that for his sister, and bought her a grand piano. And he claims he owns the company he works for, and dad knows he doesn't. Dad just listens and laughs afterwards, but it drives mother crazy; she tries to catch him up on his bragging and lies. She thought she had him once. He's always talking about his 30-acre orchard by Okanagan Lake, and then one time he said '20 acres.' Mother pounced on him with, 'You've been saying 30 acres!' He came right back with, 'Ten acres slid in the lake.' You can't trip him up."

"I guess it comes down to whether you can cope, and aren't a danger to anyone." I was quoting Dr. Gee, but I was still puzzled, in spite of all the lectures, about the vagaries of the human mind. Obsessions, delusions, depression, euphoria, suicidal impulses---how could they be explained?

"Two people can have the same tendency toward a form of mental illness," Dr. Gee intoned in his dry manner, "and some happening in one person's life will trigger that one's derangement while the other person goes along on an even keel because he hasn't been faced with the adverse condition." Causes were not recognized; boundaries remained indistinct.

Young Dr. Davidson enlightened us on Anatomy and Physiology, a difficult subject for an unmarried man to expound to 20 nubile young girls. He referred to diagrams in our text-book, and used a skeleton named Pierre to illustrate the bones of the body. Pierre was kept in a cabinet, hung on a rail arranged so that he slid out when the door was opened.

One evening the young doctor opened the cabinet and out swung Pierre dressed in a bathrobe. A wide-brimmed lady's hat trimmed with a waving feather sat jauntily on his grinning skull, and his bony feet showed through the straps of evening sandals. An umbrella hung over one arm and white gloves had been put over his dangling fingers.

Dr. Davidson was a good sport. "I see Pierre is dressed for an evening off. I trust he will be back to bare bones for my next lecture. We will go on to the muscles..." I don't know who dressed Pierre for our amusement, but we were able to go ahead with the lecture on bones the next week for his finery had all disappeared.

Materia Medica from Dr. J. M. Jackson was straight memorization, as was Bacteriology from Dr. U.P. Byrne. Dr. Jackson gave all the X-Rays to patients and nurses. A report for the years 1944-45 states that 2,900 chest X-Rays were taken, and that tuberculin tests showed a high incidence of infection in the student nurses. We were not aware of this in the early 30s, though we were sent for yearly X-Rays then, too.

Bacteriology was of more interest than the names of drugs and the dosages to be given, though Dr. Byrne lectured at such speed that I usually had four to six closely-written pages of notes after each session. Dr. Byrne worked in the basement of the Female Chronic building, in the Laboratory, and we were required to attend autopsies which he conducted there.

For such a traumatic experience the approach to post-mortem viewing was extremely casual. My first time, the supervisor told me to report to the Laboratory. The door was open and I saw rows of student nurses standing around the dissecting table, with two or three doctors also standing near its foot, and a perspiring Dr. Byrne facing me from the other side of the table, bending over a dead body. He was engaged in finishing a cut he had made from the neck to the pubis, and stretching the opening so that all the contents of the trunk were exposed to view.

I moved in beside Marshall who had come down from the ward before me, and looked around. Half the nurses might be from my class, the rest were in senior classes. Miss Hicks and Miss Marlatt were present, standing slightly behind Dr. Byrne and near the head of the table. A horrible stench filled the air. At last I looked at the body. A shriveled, purple penis caught my eye, and its very indecency and grotesqueness kept it in my side vision even as I forced myself to ignore it. Dr. Davidson placed a square of cloth on the pubic region, evidently finding that desiccated organ as repulsive a sight as I did.

Dr. Byrne was proceeding methodically to hold up for our inspection the heart, lung, liver, stomach, and kidneys, explaining the composition and function of each, then carelessly dropping it on the table beside the corpse. When he was finished, he scooped them all up and dumped them back into the body, and proceeded to sew up the incision. We were dismissed.

I walked up the three flights of stairs with Marshall - the elevator was always reserved for doctors and supervisors if they were present. "He dumped everything in any old way," I burst out when the stairwell door banged shut behind us.

"Did you expect him to take time to put things back where he found them?" asked sensible Marshall. "He sweated there for over an hour, anyway, and what difference does it make?" I had to agree, but it just didn't seem right.

I had another complaint. "That awful smell! Couldn't the autopsy be done sooner after death? That man must have died a week ago!"

"Now that's where you're wrong," said Marshall dryly. "You can bet that body is buried as soon as possible. Look at it this way, Lehman. You learned a lot there today, didn't you? I've been to four other post mortems and I learn more from each one I go to. But I always stand on the same side as Dr. Byrne. Did you notice the fan is behind him so it blows the smell away from him? That's probably why Hammond had to go out; she was right in the path of it. I know it was bad enough where we were, but it could be worse."

I attended five autopsies during my training. As Marshall said, there was something to be learned from each one. Seeing the brain exposed showed me that nerves are real. I walked in to see what appeared to be a black mustache prove to be the scalp pulled down so that the hair of the head showed around the edge just where a mustache would be. Horrible! But that lesson was an invaluable one.

"And these are the nerves that supply the eyes," Dr. Byrne drew out two thick, white, rope-like sinews. Nerves! I had thought nerves were imaginary as in "It's just nerves" or "I feel so nervous tonight." There they were, large, and solid. Dr. Davidson added to the knowledge I gained from the autopsy, in his lectures.

"Suppose you touch a hot surface," he said. "You say, 'Ouch!' and you pull your hand away. Fast. Yet the nerves in your hand have carried a message to your brain, 'That's hot!' and your brain has sent back the message, along the nerves, 'Pull your hand away, then.' At the same time, and you know how instantaneous it is, another nerve is carrying a message to your speech centre which makes you say, 'Ouch.' Without nerves, you'd burn severely."

Yes, nerves are real; as real as telegraph wires.

Miss Hicks and her staff were also lecturing the nursing classes on proper procedures. Miss Hicks laid down the rules of conduct in Ethics and included good grooming and health practices which she herself exemplified to perfection. Her own shoulders uncompromisingly straight as usual, she looked at us gravely and said, "Good posture is essential at all times, but it can be overdone. It is not necessary to be rigid. You can relax and yet keep your shoulders straight." It was difficult not to look at Oliver, who must have been the target of her instruction. Yet Oliver did not change.

"She must have been lectured about her posture from an early age," Hammond remarked, "and her exaggerated response has become a habit she can't break." She suddenly grinned. "What do you know? I'm analyzing Oliver!"

Miss Hicks must have known that many women believed we should not have a bath while menstruating. She told us, "You may have been told not to bathe during your period. There is no harm in it at all. In fact it is doubly necessary to bathe at that time, to keep clean. Nurses must have a bath every day."

Nursing Methods were given by Miss Parsons, a registered nurse. Miss Hicks and Miss Marlatt were present at these sessions too, helping to supervise our practice periods. Whether we would ever use these procedures or not, we learned, perforce, the correct way to strip and air a bed, how to make a bed with the patient in it - a full-sized rubber manikin we called 'Jenny' being more patient than a real patient, how to make a cradle bed and an ether bed. Jenny survived our clumsiness when we gave her a bed-bath, changing the rubber sheet and draw-sheet according to strict instructions and under the eagle eyes of the three RNs. We had to demonstrate the care of a sick person's teeth and mouth, care of the back, a bed shampoo, lifting a heavy patient or a helpless patient, lifting a patient to a sitting position, and even changing a mattress. Giving and removing a bedpan was fortunately easy with 'Jenny', as the pan was as clean coming out of the bed as going in.

Although bed patients on the wards were few and far between, the knowledge that there was a Female Infirmary in our building, in the same location on the second floor as ward J on the third and the large patient's dining room on the first floor - at the center back - made all this information worthwhile. We learned how to fill and apply a hot water bottle and an ice-cap, when to use an air cushion, and how to care for rubber gloves. Surely we would never have occasion to prepare (or give, perish the thought) all the kinds of enemas we had to learn to make: soapsuds, nutritive, turpentine, normal saline and whiskey enema, stimulating coffee enema, emollient, purgative, enteroclysis and proctoclysis enemas. We might not have to give them, but we did have to write an examination paper on them.

Lectures and study took care of any extra time we had after our 12 hours on the wards, but the picture changed when half of the junior class was assigned to night duty. Gladwin and I were among them.

CHAPTER SEVEN

Our dining room was buzzing with news of staff changes. "You're on F3 nights, Lehman," said Gladwin. "I saw your name on the new roster. And Langley tells me I'll be on H4 nights, so we change shifts together, at least."

"Who am I on with?" I asked. "Anyone I know?"

"You're on with Dawson," I was told. I had worked with peppy little Dawson on my first ward, and I was pleased. Gladwin was gloomy. I knew she wasn't happy about seeing less of Don, her boyfriend. Lectures would be continuing as usual which meant we'd have to be there on a night off, willy nilly. We didn't get more than one week-end off, on days or nights, each month.

We talked about our new assignments after we'd gone to bed that night. "I'm not looking forward to HR," Gladwin's voice came out of the darkness. "Langley's been there on days and she told me there are two women who've teamed up and they're both bad actors. They've been whispering and looking at the nurses as if they're planning something, and when they march down the hall together to meals nobody had better be in their way. They're both tall, one big and burly and the other thin and wiry, and they're both known as fighters. Sounds like trouble!"

"I've never seen patients team up like that." I agreed with her that it was cause for concern. "You know, I was on the bus going into town and it stopped at the penitentiary to pick up a couple of guards. They sat in the seat in front of me and it was as if they knew I worked at Essondale - but they couldn't have. I wasn't in uniform. Anyway they talked about the tough guys they had to deal with, and then one of them said, 'At least they're not crazy. I'd rather work here than out with the loonies at Essondale.' And I thought to myself, 'Yes, but ours don't gang up together like convicts sometimes do, and stage a hostage-taking riot.' You've been on the ward I'm going to. What are F3 patients like? I've sort of picked up the idea they're pretty tricky. Do they team up?"

"Not while I've been there," Gladwin stated emphatically. "They are sharper than the bottom floor wards, but each one is wrapped up in herself, like everyone else here. When they squabble they're fierce. But there's always patients who'll do the ward work, like every other ward. They're pretty good, usually."

There was silence for a few minutes and then I confided a thought that kept recurring in my mind after being locked in the side-room by Mrs. Abbott.

"I wonder how long I'd have been stuck in that room if Mrs. Abbott had really wanted to commit suicide and had hidden away under a bed or somewhere until she bled to death."

"That's what F3 is known as," exclaimed Gladwin. "The suicide ward! Not that anyone has committed suicide while I've been there, but they've threatened to do themselves in. I've heard that there's been a suicide there and the nurse held responsible was fired. But no one's been fired since we've been here, have they?"

"I don't know how they decide where to place the patients," I speculated. "Mrs. Abbott sounds like a third floor patient yet she's on F4. Maybe because she's violent enough when she goes off and F3 doesn't have side-rooms. Or maybe she has TB..."

"Well, I wouldn't worry about it, Lehman. There's some friendly women on F3. You'll like Mrs. Cook. She's like a mother to the nurses. You'd wonder why she's in the hospital at all." The room became quiet and we dropped off to sleep.

We started night shift on the first of the month. The days were getting shorter as winter approached and it was strange going on duty in the deepening dusk, at the hour we had been accustomed to finish work. We had worked the day before, and slept that night, so our attempts to get some sleep that day had not been very successful. I was keyed up to meet this new challenge.

Dawson's pixie face and insouciant air were familiar and calming as she led the way into the office where the day staff was assembled for the report, which was read by the Charge Nurse, Miss

Seymour. The rest of us waited while Seymour and Dawson made the count.

The two nurses formed a striking contrast as they moved around the two dayrooms. Solid, imposing Seymour sailed along like a massive warship with pert little Dawson, the escort vessel bouncing along beside her. Everyone was accounted for, and the day nurses went off to leave the ward in our care.

Bedspreads had been removed and blinds drawn down before the supper hour, so that bedtime preparations could begin soon after our arrival. All the patients had to be out of the dayrooms by 7:30, with lights out an hour later. Blue lights were switched on in the dormitories so that we could make out the forms of the sleeping patients through the corridor windows on our hourly checks, a task that fell to me as the junior nurse.

Mrs. Cook came to our aid in learning the vagaries of the women who did not attend to their own bedtime routine. Mrs. Cook was all that Gladwin had promised, a warm, motherly woman whose own eccentricities were not apparent to me.

"You'll have to see that Mrs. Field is made to wash and she'll never undress without prodding. Most of the ones who need help are in this room and the next. They have to be helped to get up again in the morning. There's women who'll help dress them, though."

She drew our attention to a patient who was filling an enema bag. "Mind Mrs. Crestwell there. She'll sit on the toilet for an hour with that enema tube stuck into her if you let her. Has to have one every night. Says her insides turn to cement if she doesn't."

A few nights later Dawson called me over to the toilet stall where Mrs. Crestwell was administering her nightly purge. "Lehman, look here," she whispered. "She's not giving herself an enema. She's douching. Just look at the expression on her face! Bliss, pure bliss. I watched her fill the bag and she has a douche tip, not an enema tip." Dawson giggled. "If it keeps her happy....Just get her off there if you can before too long." We left Mrs. Crestwell to her self-gratifying pastime and went about our other chores.

Some of the women, the ones who needed assistance in dressing and undressing, had to be attended in the showers, though without the complete involvement necessary with the catatonics on the floor above. There, as here, I marvelled at the many different body builds - any firm that can advertise 'One size fits all' should spend some time in a women's shower room. All sizes, all shapes. And the variations in shape as well as size were an exercise in permutations and combinations. It was a revelation to me to see that perfect proportions might be seen in different sizes. The lack of exercise in the mental hospital led to more imperfections than perfections, though.

I studied the hermaphrodite with interest. She was surly, which might be expected, and I was careful not to stare. Her manly chest and strong arms were evidence of greater than normal strength.

My first experience with an epileptic was frightening for I had no warning and no instruction. An apparition in white - she was in her nightgown - came toward me with arms outstretched, her fingers clawing the air convulsively, and her mouth contorted. Spittle was forming around her lips as she stuttered unintelligibly. I thought she meant to attack me when in truth she was looking for help, and I backed away. She took another faltering step, then fell to the floor where she shook uncontrollably. I was unable to move, horrified.

Dawson arrived, fetched by a patient. She knelt beside the unfortunate woman and turned her on her side, calmly putting her key between the woman's teeth as the jerking continued. The convulsions gradually lessened, then stopped, and the patient's eyes held a dazed expression.

"Help me get her to her feet, Lehman. She's wet herself. Take her to the washroom and help her clean up. I'll bring a clean gown. Be careful, she's not right out of it yet."

By the time we learned about epilepsy in our lectures, as it was understood in the 1930's, I had accepted the condition as calmly as Dawson and was able to insert my key between the teeth as she had done. In later years this practice was discontinued as being unnecessary and possibly injurious to the teeth.

That epileptics exhibited such frustration and rage at being classed as mental patients is not surprising, before the drugs that control the seizures were discovered. Unfortunately the stigma associated with the incorrect diagnosis affects the 400,000 Canadians that have epilepsy today. It still comes as a surprise to many people to learn that epilepsy is not linked to mental illness, low I.Q., or violence, beliefs held even by the medical profession until it was discovered that epilepsy is caused by a brief malfunction of the brain's electrical system. Otherwise the person affected is perfectly normal, and certainly not of low intelligence.

In some cases surgery is effective, in the relatively small number of cases in which the place in the brain where the seizure begins can be identified and removed without impairment of other functions. The greatest improvement that can be made is that people become educated about this 'seizure disorder,' and learn to accept the afflicted person as they would any physically handicapped individual.

Though a relief nurse was provided - one of the two night nurses on the bottom floor wards - for the top floor wards, on our ward Dawson was alone while I went to lectures or midnight meal, and I was alone while she was away. There was no phone other than in the office, and no alarm system to call for help from the dormitories. Yet I felt secure in the knowledge that not only Mrs. Cook, but some of the other 'good' patients would come to my help if necessary. Mentally ill persons live in a private world created by their particular delusions and their battles are fought mainly in their own minds.

"I can't go to sleep this early," Mrs. Cook would say as she joined Dawson and me at our table after the dormitory lights were turned off. She settled back into the extra chair she had brought in from the rotunda. "Now don't worry about rules," she said the first night. "If I hear a key in the door I'll just walk back to my room and I've been to the bathroom, see? There's no need to upset the Night Supervisor." With several monotonous hours ahead of us, we welcomed her company, especially for the time when one of us was away and the other was left alone.

Miss Windermere did not drop in unexpectedly very often, but she was certain to accompany the doctor when he made rounds, at any time from nine to midnight. They usually appeared before ten so that drugs could be ordered for any patient who was keeping the others awake. When the doctor's visit was over, the ward quiet and dark, we settled down to hours of reading or studying and trying to stay awake.

Hourly checks of the sleeping patients had to be made and this helped me to rouse myself from the soporific effect of books - especially text-books. Being on nights was certainly an advantage for studying, and I brought books from the library in town as I was an avid reader. But I had to find something to do that would help to pass the long hours.

"Bring some wool and knitting needles, and a sweater pattern," Mrs. Cook said. "Can you knit at all? I'll help you with the pattern." I was pleased with the suggestion and brought the materials with me after my next night off.

Mrs. Cook watched me casting on stitches, awkwardly handling the unaccustomed needles. I hadn't knitted anything more intricate than a scarf, and that was years before.

"Here, let me show you," she said, taking the needles from me and pulling out the uneven mess. Holding the two needles together, she twisted and looped a beautiful firm edge, which I eventually mastered under her guidance. Mrs. Cook was a competent knitter and thanks to her patient teaching I made all the knitted articles I could use. I then needed another diversion and she suggested crocheting.

"You can make doilies and edgings for tablecloths and pillow cases," she said, "for your hope chest." My 'hope' chest was my bottom drawer, as it was for most of the girls of that era. The 'hope' part was the hope of marriage, if we could meet a man able to support a wife and family. For a woman to work after marriage was unthinkable. You would be taking work from the family provider.

Thanks to the five or six night shifts during my three years at the hospital, and a gift from the girls in my class when I was leaving after graduation to be married, I had a full cedar chest with sets of the items Mrs. Cook had mentioned in it, plus two top sheets with three-inch inserts of patterned crocheted lace at the hem and matching pillow slip edgings. I was also wearing at my wedding a pair of lacy crocheted gloves that I had made on night duty. When I was complimented on any of these accomplishments I took great pleasure in saying, "I was taught how to knit and crochet by a patient at Essondale," knowing the incredulity this statement produced. I wouldn't have believed it myself, before I worked there.

Toward the end of my time on her ward Mrs. Cook stopped coming out to sit with us, and we missed her company. I hoped I wouldn't see her go 'off' and I didn't, for she only stayed remote and moody, and irritable. I remember her fondly as a good friend who added a new dimension to my life.

While I was determined to stay awake all night, Dawson had no such compulsion. She was able to cat-nap, resting her head on her hand with her elbow on the table and a book on her lap. The least noise brought her awake, and with the rattle of a key in the lock she opened her eyes and gave the appearance of having been absorbed in her book as we rose to our feet for the visit of the Night Supervisor.

Miss Windermere was a handsome middle-aged registered nurse who gave the impression something was missing from her life. And that 'something' was a man.

"Isn't it sickening the way she fawns over the doctors!" Dawson exclaimed one night after Miss Windermere had fluttered out after the doctor on duty. Doctors always preceded nurses but there was a flirtatious air to the Night Supervisor's servility, and often an uncomfortable awareness on the good doctor's part could be sensed.

One evening Miss Windermere attempted a curious playfulness with a new young doctor who was taking psychiatric training at the hospital. Her frivolous actions surprised us.

The dormitory door opened that night at the time we were expecting rounds to be made, and Miss Windermere popped in by herself. She hissed, "Don't tell Dr. Barlow I'm here!" and stood against the wall so that she wouldn't be seen when he opened the door. How she got ahead of him without being noticed was a mystery, for he came in so closely on her heels that she hadn't yet seen our foolish expressions as we stood in her presence, as required, giving the game away.

The young doctor strode in saying, "I couldn't find Miss Windermere...What in the blazes is wrong with you two? What's the joke, I'd like to know?" We were trying not to giggle, unable to speak.

Miss Windermere came out of the corner trying to put a good face on her foolishness, and looking daggers at us for not playing the game. "I was only playing a joke on you," she began, but Dr. Barlow was coldly furious.

"Do you need any sedatives?" he asked Dawson curtly, ignoring the Supervisor. At Dawson's shake of the head he turned and stalked out, with Miss Windermere scurrying at his heels, her color high.

Dawson and I collapsed into our chairs and laughed until we choked in our attempt to be quiet. "There's life in the old girl yet," Dawson spluttered when she recovered her voice. "I wonder just what games she thought he would play?"

In the meantime Gladwin was finding that H4, a top floor ward, was proving to be not as bad as she had first feared. We were rinsing out our stockings and undies and cleaning our white shoes in the mornings before going to bed and trying to sleep in our darkened room.

"Nights are sure different from days," Gladwin remarked. "I can't get over how busy we are for the few hours just after we go on duty, and in the mornings before we go off the ward, and how quiet the ward is in between."

"Any trouble with the patients on H4?" I inquired. This top floor ward was known for almost as many calls 'Help on H4!' as there were for 'Help on J!'.

"Nothing we can't control with sedatives," Gladwin said. "Even the two chums that were pals are cooling off. I wouldn't have believed how quiet the ward is all night."

"The same on F3!" I exclaimed. "Only we don't have many that need an extra sedative to what they get from the day staff. But isn't it scary sitting in the dormitory corridor with a hundred unstable women around you? It's bad enough on F3."

"Oh, we don't sit in the dormitory on H4," Gladwin explained. "We set up a table in the rotunda with the dormitory door open, so we're not far from the phone. And there's always two of us on the top floor wards at night. I don't know if I'd like being alone like you are, even on the better wards."

"It's surprising what you get used to," I answered. What was the opposite of the saying, "The grass always looks greener on the other side of the fence?" Not to a psychiatric nurse; what had seemed terrifying at first turned out to be bearable, in the end. Even enjoyable at times.

"Let's hope we can get some sleep today," Gladwin said, as we got into our beds. "We sure have a lot of traffic by our room."

We had congratulated ourselves on being given a room right across from the shower room and the toilets, a location that proved to be a distinct disadvantage on nights. We never seemed to get enough sleep.

We were supposed to sleep from eight in the morning until three in the afternoon, and the day Home Supervisor frowned upon anyone appearing out of her room between those hours. But those were the hours the Home was cleaned and polished by women who were brought over from the good wards. For them it made a pleasant change from the dayrooms.

For us, with the utility room close by as well as the two rooms that required daily cleaning, it meant the unavoidable noise of doors being opened and closed, pails clanking and mops being wrung out, clanking against the bucket, plus the traffic back and forth outside our room as the tasks were accomplished.

Even the 'good' patients became unreliable at times as their inner demons took over. Usually the signs were there for the nurses to recognize and remove the woman from her work until she settled down again, but it was my misfortune to discover the evidence of imminent breakdown in the Home one afternoon.

On awakening from a fitful sleep I went across to the shower room planning to take a warm bath to refresh myself before getting dressed. "Personal hydrotherapy," I said to myself. "If it's good for the patients it must be good for the nurse."

The washrooms were sparkling clean and I expected to find a shining tub, as usual. Instead I came upon a disgusting sight. A huge pile of stinking feces rose to an astonishing height from the bottom of the tub. "What on earth is the matter?" asked Oliver, who was coming in for a shower. "You look positively sick." I showed her the revolting mess.

"Must have been one of the workers," Oliver stated the obvious. "Probably in revolt against the authority we represent. Her dementia will be noticed on the ward and she won't be coming over for awhile. Some other poor soul will have to clean this up." Calmly she stepped into a shower stall and I decided a shower would do me that day too. I wouldn't even look at that tub for days to come.

Getting enough sleep was always a problem, and nurses came off a night shift which could be six months long with hollow eyes. Just when our systems were adjusting to sleeping in the daytime, we had one or sometimes two nights off, when we joined the regular world and went to bed at the regular time. A night off was really two days off and one good night's sleep. It also meant coming back to a 12-hour shift after a day without sleep.

Along with insufficient sleep, we were subjected to an erratic system of meals. Eating breakfast before going to bed was as unnatural as having supper upon awakening from sleep. We found it easy to skip one or both of these meals and supplement our midnight dinner with snacks in the kitchen of the Nurses' Home. There was a Tuck Shoppe only a few steps from the Home which was very convenient. All in all night shift made for a topsy-turvy life.

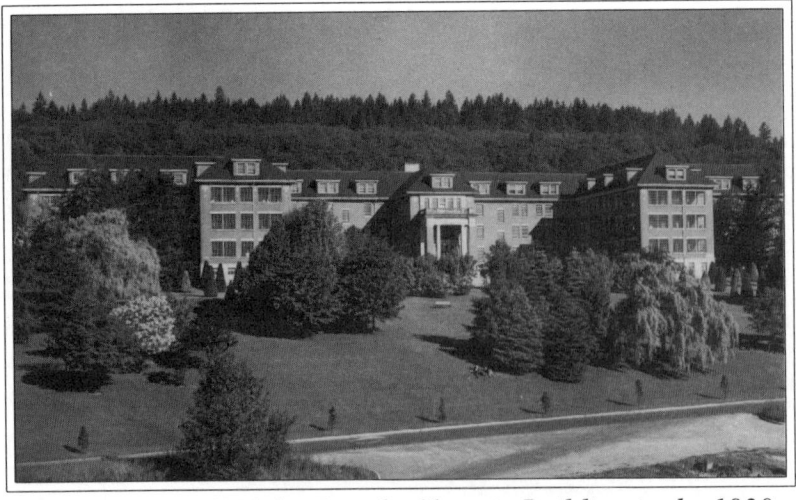

East Lawn - called the Female Chronic Building in the 1930s.

CHAPTER EIGHT

In many ways night shifts were lonely intervals in our lives. I missed the camaraderie of meal-times. The half-hour allowed for our one meal on nights, at midnight, was a hurried affair. Except for the top floor wards, our absence meant that one person was alone with 100 patients, and we just ate and returned to the ward. Sitting outside on the front steps as we did on days was out.

It was through Marshall, the super-efficient senior I had worked with on F4, that the daylight hours after three o'clock became time for getting out in the fresh air to explore the surrounding countryside.

The days were still warm though the nights were getting colder. Autumn was turning the leaves to beautiful yellows and oranges, with vine maples a brilliant red amongst the various greens of the underbrush common to our coastal forests. We had only to cross the railway tracks at the bottom of the hill to be in the uncleared area on our side of the Coquitlam River, a short distance to the Red Bridge. Occasional farms on the other side gave way to the outlying streets and homes of the City of Port Coquitlam, with its one main street.

Marshall had been at the hospital two years before Gladwin and me, and with the lack of other entertainment due to its remote location, had become a great walker. She liked company and chased up any of the night staff who would join her on her walks.

"C'mon, you two! Time to get up and get some exercise!" was meant to rouse Gladwin and me from our lazy beds at the permitted hour of three.

"Where are we going?" I asked, yawning. I could have slept another couple of hours. Gladwin turned over with a sluggish, "Have a heart, Marshall. I was off yesterday and I need more sleep."

"Give me ten minutes, Marshall. I do need some exercise," I agreed. I got up and dressed in a hurry.

Marshall and Hammond were waiting for me and Marshall took us out the back door of the Home. A path led up the cleared hillside, past some houses which Marshall said were for the supplementary staff. "That one is where the head gardener lives," she pointed out. They were neatly fenced in and men who were obviously patients, by their institutional clothes, were cleaning up the gardens for the winter. They leaned on their hoes to watch us go by. Marshall spoke to them or nodded a greeting. "There's the head gardener," she said, waving to Mr. Renton who was in charge of the workers.

Halfway up the hill we came to the firehall. Two firemen lounged on a bench, their cleaning and polishing done for the day. Marshall stopped for a chat.

"Any fires lately?" Marshall asked, after introducing Hammond and me.

"Nope, but we're always ready," one of the men said. "With the patients being allowed to smoke, it's always a chance."

"Oh, they can't light a cigarette without being under our supervision," Marshall answered. "They have to ask for a match, and they have to stay out in the rotunda or on the porch, with a nurse right with them. I guess it's the same with the men."

"As long as you all know you do have to stay with them," the fireman said. "And as long as some visitor doesn't give a patient a box of matches. Or even one match." They had a good job, but knew the dangerous possibilities in such a place. One firetruck was all they had, and there was no other closer than Port Coquitlam, which was manned by volunteer firemen who had to be called in from wherever they were.

After a few minutes' chat we turned to go, and the older man said with a twinkle in his eye, "We have the pole all shined up for you. Go ahead and take your friends in, Marshall. I know you want to."

"Great fun," we said, after wrapping our arms and legs around the pole and dropping down from the second floor a couple of times. "We'll come again!" Saying good-bye to the men, we started toward the back of the three institutional buildings.

"Do you ever go up to the woods?" Hammond asked. "It's not far, and there's probably paths through them."

"No, I don't," Marshall said firmly. "And we're not going to. There are paths, all right. The male patients with grounds privileges go on up to some lakes back there, and I'd love to see them myself. But can you imagine meeting a patient in the woods?" She shuddered.

"Why should the men get all the breaks?" Hammond asked heatedly. "There's a lot of outdoor work for the men, too. It's not fair!"

"Hammond, you know the women can't be out on their own here. They'd be fair game for the men on the grounds; and maybe some women wouldn't mind." Marshall chuckled.

"Well, they could take turns," Hammond insisted. "Keep all the men in and let the women out on alternate days."

We were now behind the Female Chronic Building and I was studying the windows on the top floor, trying to pick out the one I had been looking out of when I was shut in the side-room. There wasn't a soul in sight. If I had yelled nobody would have heard me.

We went by some tennis courts. "These don't look as if they're used very often," I said. "I haven't heard anyone talk about playing a game, even in the summer."

"The day staff's too tired at the end of their shift, and they've been on their feet most of the time," Marshall said. "And not enough of the staff own a racquet, anyway. No one, that I know. It's a game for people who have time, and money. Do you two know anything about tennis?" We didn't. "If I ever get a chance to borrow a couple of racquets and some balls, we'll get out and bat the ball around, anyway," Marshall said, leading us around the buildings to the driveway in front which led back to the Nurses' Home.

The walks instigated by Marshall were refreshing for cobwebby minds and I never turned her down when she came asking for me. Gladwin, for all her love of the outdoors, went into town every chance she got, and was always tired on days she slept in the Home. I suspected she was getting quite serious about Don. I had met him briefly and liked him.

A few days later Marshall and I crossed the Red Bridge and

headed for Port Coquitlam. We passed some scattered small farms, then four or five blocks of houses from the schoolhouse to the center of town. There was a grocery store, a hotel, two restaurants, and some smaller establishments stretching the two blocks to the railway line that marked the end of the main street. There was a harness shop and a blacksmith down a side street, and a fairly new set of gas pumps to service the automobiles that had been bought in the good times before the Depression, in the 'Roaring Twenties'.

A large, red-brick city hall set in landscaped grounds drew my attention. "How come they call this burg a city?" I wondered aloud.

"That goes back to the time they thought this would be the terminus of the Canadian Pacific Railway," Marshall told me. "Just like Port Moody was expected to be the terminus of the Canadian National when that railway was built." Port Moody was the town at the end of Burrard Inlet, not far from Port Coquitlam. "Though that was 40 years before the boom hit here. In both cases lots were selling for a thousand dollars each, and I'd be surprised if they cost more than a couple of hundred today. The balloon burst when the CNR continued on to Hastings Mill further down the inlet, where the city of Vancouver is now. The same thing happened with Port Coquitlam. The CPR chose Vancouver for its terminus. You wonder how these rumors start," She frowned.

A train was crossing the roadway in front of us, and it stopped, then began to back up. "What on earth!" I exclaimed. "That train is blocking the roadway, and now it's backing up!" There was one automobile waiting on this side, a square-backed Ford with side curtains in which the cellophane windows were cracked and patched over with strips of cloth.

"We'll start back," Marshall said. "The railway yards extend to both sides of the road, and the trains shunt back and forth for as long as they please." She laughed. "It makes a good excuse for the nurses who come in late, as long as they don't try it too often. They just say they were held up by a train in Port Coquitlam."

We were passing the good-sized hotel on the main street. "This is a popular place with some of the nurses," Marshall remarked, "It has a beer parlor. And there's another one about half a mile over the tracks, and one at the Pitt River bridge. I can't understand anyone wasting time in a beer parlor, can you?"

Then she laughed. "I hear that when the nurses and attendants get loosened up they mimic the patients, reaching for the ceiling and jumping over imaginary wires, and repeating some of the crazy things the patients say."

"I don't think many of our class spend time in beer parlors," I said, troubled. Nurses wouldn't have a good reputation in Coquitlam, I thought. Richmond had told me that teachers could get fired if they were seen in a beer parlor. It just wasn't socially acceptable.

"It only takes a few bad apples to spoil a bushel," Marshall said in her cheerful voice. The frown on Marshall's forehead wasn't a sign of a glum disposition, for though she had a serious nature, her voice revealed a zest for living. I had great admiration for Marshall.

Oliver came along on our first visit to Colony Farm. This walk became a favorite with us. An impressive entrance road with shade trees along one side of it led from the main road to the buildings near the river. We passed these and crossed by a wooden bridge to the dike on the other side of Coquitlam River. A path along the top of the dike took us to the Red Bridge, and as the serpentine windings of the river took it much closer to the main road at this point, we had only a short walk up to the Nurses' Home.

Colony Farm was always of interest, as there were horses and cows, pigs and sheep in the fields. The farm was managed by experts who made it a showplace, and raised the best breeds in all categories of livestock. The animals were prize winners in agricultural fairs in the Pacific Northwest as well as across Canada.

"I've seen Colony Farm exhibits at the PNE", Oliver said. "Whole rows of big fat cows, 'Colony Farm Bess' and 'Colony Farm Flossie' and all with a lot of blue ribbons and Championship awards displayed in their stalls. The same with their horses, and other animals."

"The farm is a part of the hospital," Marshall told us. "It provides milk and butter, meat and vegetables for the whole place, and I understand it runs at a profit. That large square building houses the male patients who work here. The smaller one is for the attendants. The houses are for foremen and managers." There was a comfortable air of normalcy in the farm atmosphere that would be beneficial to patients who lived and worked there. There were barns and sheds and fenced-off fields where some fall plowing was being done.

I had grown up on a farm and had many pleasant memories of the freedom of fields and woodlands. "What a healthy, natural atmosphere for a patient," I said. Just then we had a whiff of the manure that was being spread on a field. "But not that kind of atmosphere," I laughed. "That's one of the reasons I'm never going to marry a farmer."

Our afternoon walks usually took less than a couple of hours and gave us an appetite for supper in the staff dining room. But even the table seating had changed with the shifts so the old comradeship of our group was missing. On our nights off we sometimes stayed out at the Home because of lectures, and when we did we were allowed to go out when we pleased. One such day Marshall and I were both off and she made plans for an outing.

"Be sure to have breakfast in the morning, Lehman. We'll start right after we change out of uniform." The fresh air was invigorating after the long hours inside and we stepped out with the energy and enthusiasm of youth and good spirits.

"Where are we going?" I inquired, as we headed for Port Coquitlam. "To the Minnekhada Ranch," Marshall answered. "It's on the Pitt River near Pitt Lake, a fair hike. It's going to take over an hour each way."

We crossed the railway tracks at the edge of town and passed the Agricultural grounds with its 'Aggie Hall' where a fall fair was held every year, and dances through the winter months. Right next to it was a hotel and beer parlor, and there Marshall turned toward the mountains. There were more blocks of houses along Prairie Road, then a scattering on Coast Meridian - we were zig-zagging our way east and north. We passed a few farms on a road that took us along a creek, so deeply set in the ground it was almost a slough.

"This is Back Ditch Road," Marshall informed me. "We're on a dike because the creek floods when the snow melts in the mountains in the spring. We're right below Burke Mountain. The ranch is at the end of this road."

"Does the creek actually rise this high?" I asked. There were only a few inches of clear water. I could see the gravel bottom.

"Depends on the snowfall," Marshall said. "It has been known to wash right over the top of the dike. There's just enough water there now for the salmon to come up and spawn. The creek will be full of spawning salmon soon. You could almost walk across on their backs. Then they die, and the stench is awful. I've been along here when the dead salmon smell to high heaven. They draw the bears, so it's not very safe to be walking. Though I guess the bears would be full already and wouldn't be hungry. But I don't trust bears."

We had been hiking for what seemed like hours and at last we came to a gate with a sign, 'Minnekhada Ranch. Private Property.'

"Less than a mile now," Marshall announced as she opened the gate and closed it behind us. "The owner won't be here in the middle of the week. He's the Lieutenant-Governor of the province and this is his weekend retreat. He brings his friends out for hunting and fishing. And probably partying," she smiled.

In a short while we could see barns and sheds and an ordinary farmhouse. A splendid lodge was under construction, with a lake nearby on which Mallard ducks and Canada geese were to be seen.

"The geese will soon be going south," Marshall noted. "Doesn't that lake look natural? It was man-made by widening a stream that runs through right here, and sloping the sides down. Pretty, isn't it?" It was attractive, bordered by birch and maple trees in their autumn colors with evergreens in the background. Green grass made a park-like setting.

The reason for Marshall's choice of this destination now became evident. Some men were working on the construction of the lodge and one of them, young and happy-go-lucky looking, came over to us. Marshall introduced Bob but he didn't have time to chat. The foreman was looking our way.

He spoke to Marshall. "So you are off tonight, Hazel. I'll pick you up at 9:30, then. See you." He nodded to me and went back to work, whistling.

"We'd better start back," Marshall said cheerfully. "I can sleep until time for lectures if I miss supper. Bob and I are going dancing tonight. He'll take me home after the dance so I won't have to come back here until tomorrow in time to go to work."

"How did you meet Bob?" I asked as we set a good pace going back.

"At a dance at the Aggie Hall. He didn't have a car then but when he got the job at Minnekhada Ranch he bought a jalopy. It gets us around, when it isn't breaking down. It was sitting in someone's yard and he got it for $35, but he had to get it running to drive it away. He's good with engines."

"Gladwin says her boyfriend's old car is always getting flat tires, and he has to patch the tubes at the side of the road."

"That, too," Marshall agreed. "I suppose he has to crank it to start, and rush back to the wheel to adjust the spark and the choke. Bob's showing me how to do it so he can crank and I can move the levers. The brakes aren't good so he uses the emergency brake to stop."

"At least the roads are not so dusty now that we've had some rain. The cars that have passed us today have raised hardly any dust at all." None of the roads were paved or macadamized. We had to walk on dirt and gravel surfaces wherever we went as there were no sidewalks. I was glad to get to bed when we got back to the Home.

Some of the other girls on nights joined us on our walks at times and the camaraderie established this way led to several invitations to each other's homes, sometimes overnight on weekends. Hammond and Oliver were frequent companions. I had told my friends that my parents were sometimes away and I didn't have a key to our house so there was no point in going home on some of my days off.

"Are your folks terribly rich, Lehman, going off on trips so often?" Oliver's pert inquiry was tempered by the gentle smile on her face.

"Hey, would I be out here if they were? They're not going on trips, just out to our farm in the Fraser Valley."

"Well, I call that rich," Hammond joined in the teasing. "Having a farm in the country and a city house, too."

"It's not a working farm right now," I explained. Dad was not a farmer, though he had tried it for 15 years. Low, low prices, like a dollar for a ten-gallon can of milk, and two dozen eggs for 15 cents forced him out. My parents had sold the animals by auction, along with all the farm implements. "We had renters for a year and then they left, and it's up for sale or rent now. Nobody's thinking of farming in these times, it seems. So my parents have all the expenses, like taxes, and no income from it. They go out to keep a check on it and cut the lawn and keep it tidy. It's a white elephant, that's what."

"I was just teasing," Oliver said. "We're both off on the weekend, aren't we? Why don't you come home with me?"

Oliver's parents lived in Vancouver. Her father was a school principal. His army service showed in his rigidly upright bearing and a cold, reserved manner maintained even in his home. He spent most of the time we were there in his study.

Mrs. Oliver—how strange it was to use my friend's name for her parents—was a large woman, so tightly corseted that she was always slightly out of breath. "Ruth, take your friend—Lehman? What is your first name? Take Eva to a movie tonight. I'll be at a Wayward Girls meeting and your father has a poker game. Clara Bow is on at the Orpheum tonight." She sighed. "That theater has such an elegant lobby! I always feel like I'm at the opera, going up those magnificent red carpeted stairs...cherubs on the ceilings...those chandeliers...the velvet curtains!" Her manner became brisk. "I have to go, girls. A committee meeting on Ways and Means. I'm supplying the refreshments and I must rush and pick them up at the delicatessen." She put on a wide-brimmed hat trimmed lavishly with artificial flowers, smoothed on kid gloves, picked up a light coat and purse, and was gone.

"What do you think, Lehman?" Oliver asked. "Shall we have a sleep now and go to the movie tonight, or would you like to go to Stanley Park?"

"Oh, Stanley Park! It's too nice out to waste the day sleeping! I've only been around the park once in a car. There's a zoo, isn't there?" We caught a streetcar and got off at the park entrance, and walked in to the zoo, where we treated ourselves to a hot dog and watched the antics of the monkeys. Then we passed the duck pond and crossed to Lumberman's Arch and sat on the grass, watching the harbor traffic. The completely forested North Shore mountains rose to snow-tipped heights on the other side of Burrard Inlet, a familiar sight to Oliver but wondrous to me.

"Can you make out the Lions, just a bit to the right?" Oliver pointed out the distinguishing features, the heavy mane and large head of one, and the sleeker female outline of the other recumbent shape at the very crest of the range. "And farther to the right is Grouse Mountain. There's a road up to the lodge on Grouse. We drive up for Sunday dinner sometimes. I love the view of the city from the top." She pointed out the ferry that crossed the inlet, and the CPR ferry came through First Narrows from Vancouver Island just before we had to leave. Large freighters took on loads at the industries on the waterfront across from us, and tugboats towing booms of logs brought them in to the saw-mill holding areas. It was all new to me, and I hated to leave. Weariness was overtaking us, though, and we knew there would be no movie that night.

Busy with her meetings, Mrs. Oliver did no cooking of meals while I was there. That evening there was a plate of left-over dainty sandwiches and one of a picked over mixture of small cakes with sweet fillings, set out on the bare kitchen table, for our supper. A paper bag of doughnuts had been added. Mrs. Oliver poured tea.

"Help yourselves, now. Your father has already gone out, and I have a dinner meeting at seven. I just have time for a cup of tea."

In the morning there were two bags on the table, the doughnuts and some breakfast rolls. Neither parent was around. Oliver and I took the early bus back to Essondale.

One day Gladwin and I decided to walk into New Westminster, to her home. "We live at this end of town," she said. "It'll be about five miles, peanuts after your hike to Minnekhada and back. We won't have to walk back. Don will drive us." I had ridden in Don's old car, the joy of his life. The radiator leaked and he carried a can to get water from streams near the road when it started to heat up. There were three pedals on the floor - low gear, reverse, and brake. The cellophane in the side curtains was yellow and cracked, as it was on all old cars. The gas tank was under the front seat, so Gladwin and I had to get out when he needed gas.

Gladwin told me about her family on the walk into town. "Dad died when we all had the 'flu, after the war," she said. "It must have been awful for Mother, as he was the first to get it, and she couldn't even go to his funeral because she and I had the 'flu next, at the same time. And Dave was small, he got it next. I remember how sick I was - I was about eight years old. Couldn't eat a thing for days. Then the first thing I wanted was a piece of cake. It tasted like sand! I'll never forget it. I know now it was my mouth that was like sand."

Mrs. Gladwin was a spare, hollow-cheeked, worn-looking woman who supported herself and her family by taking in washing. She was ironing. "The ironing board is never put away," my roommate told me. Though her tiredness showed in the stoop of her shoulders as she pushed her hair out of her eyes with one hand while she kept the iron moving with the other, Gladwin's mother greeted us warmly. "It's good to meet you, Lehman." She used her daughter's name for me unselfconsciously. "No, Myrtle, you're not to help me. You've had a long walk and you've been up all night. Get yourselves a snack and you'd better sleep for a few hours. Will Don be taking you back?" I felt very much at home at Gladwin's, and the two of us managed to help Mrs. Gladwin for a few hours before we left that evening.

Marshall's home was only half a mile from mine, I discovered when she took me home. Her frown was deeper than usual when she opened the door, to be almost knocked off her feet by a chubby girl of indeterminate age who hurled herself against her, babbling "Hazie, Hazie," while she hugged her sister and gave her moist kisses. She had protruding slanted eyes in a round face and the thick, inarticulate speech of a Mongoloid. "Take it easy, sweetie," my friend said, disentangling herself as we entered the room. "Say hello to my friend Lehman. This is my sister, Grace," she said quietly to me.

The young girl - or was she a young woman? - stroked my arm affectionately. Her hand felt dry and scratchy. Mrs. Marshall came in at that moment, producing a handkerchief to wipe Grace's nose, which ran continually. "Please excuse Gracie," she said while giving her a doll to hug. "She can't help it; her nose is a nuisance. The doctor can't do anything for it." She was as easygoing as Marshall was resolute. I was impressed by their shared love for the child of misfortune in the family.

"Okay, let's decide where we're going to sleep tonight," Marshall took charge. "There's no one at home at your place, you said. Let's go and see if we can get in. There might be a window open." On the way over she explained, "Grace and I could sleep together, but you'd have to sleep on the couch. There'd be no need if we can get into your house."

We tried the doors at my place, then the windows that we could reach. The easiest one to enter, off the porch, proved to be unlocked, and slid open without effort. "Good," said Marshall. "We'll get our things and sleep here."

We were there when my parents arrived home the next day. "The window was unfastened?" Mother fretted, while Dad went to check the lock. "It's a good thing it was you girls who found it and not a burglar. We never locked a door on the farm, but here in the city...there's so many people around."

Dad went off to the house he was building - he was happily back in his former occupation - and mother made cinnamon buns for us. "Take some back with you for snacks," she urged. "I'm sure your meals are wrong way around on nights and the buns will do for breakfast or supper."

"Did you get a key?" Marshall asked me on the bus going back.

"They don't have an extra key," I answered. "And mother won't leave one under the mat. I guess you don't need one." I was thinking of Grace.

"Right. Mother's always home." Yes, she would be.

One afternoon, Hammond and I were in her room studying for an exam in Bacteriology, a tough subject. Oliver was away and Gladwin, as usual, was catching up on sleep. We were asking each other questions and checking answers, when Hammond lay back on the bed and exclaimed, "November is the worst month of the year!" It was teaming rain outside.

"The rains sure cut into our walks," I responded, glad to take a break. I laughed, "Except when Marshall decides we're going anyway. She waxed my shoes with floor polish yesterday when I said it was too wet to go out. And it was okay, at that. Just a Scotch mist. But it's pouring today."

"Maybe we'll get snow for Christmas." Hammond's face was

forlorn. "I guess I'll have to go home sometime in Christmas week. We're not likely to get Christmas Eve or the next night off, and I don't care!"

"Oh, Hammond, why not?" I felt that she wanted to talk yet I sensed an unhappiness that I really didn't want to hear about.

"I don't even go home on most of my nights off," Hammond had turned over on her bed so that her face was buried in her arms which were folded over the pillow.

"You don't?" I said weakly. This was outside of my perception of family. Feeling very inadequate I ventured to ask, "What do you do then?" I was sure Oliver would have known if her roommate stayed at the Home on her nights off.

Hammond turned her face toward me, her fine blond hair falling partly over her woeful expression. "Oh, I go into town and walk around the stores, and maybe go to a movie. I've been home with Oliver and I know she wonders why I don't ask her to mine. But I just can't tell her; we're too close here. I couldn't stand her sympathy every hour of the day, even if she wasn't saying anything."

I felt guilty. I had taken Gladwin and Oliver and Marshall home with me when my parents weren't away, but I hadn't thought of Hammond. She maintained a self-sufficient air which discouraged confidences. She was breaking all her rules today as she went on, tears starting to spill out of her eyes, "It's not so bad on nights. My mother knows I have to be here for lectures so she doesn't expect me to get home on my nights off. But we'll likely be going on days after Christmas - oh! I don't know what to do!" Her face hidden again, she rolled back and forth, sobbing.

I didn't know what to do. I drew my knees up to my chin, sitting on Oliver's bed, and wished I were anywhere but here. I had to say something, so I ventured a tentative, "What's the matter, Hammond?"

The unhappy girl sat up to reach for a handkerchief to wipe her eyes and blow her nose. "It's my f-f-father!" she shuddered. "I have an awful time, getting him to leave me alone!" She stretched out again, facing me, her handkerchief held to her eyes.

"But, your mother -? Doesn't she know?" I was horror-stricken at this sordid revelation, and heartsick for my friend.

"She goes into her own room and locks the door." Hammond's voice was choked with the tears she was trying to hold back.

"Can't you tell her?" This was something I had never imagined, that a girl wasn't safe from her own father.

"I've tried!" There was pure agony in her exclamation. "She just turns away and won't listen! Oh, Lehman, I feel so dirty!"

I jumped off the bed and sat beside her, drawing her up for a hug. "You're not dirty! You're one of the nicest people I know." I was crying too. "I wouldn't go home at all if..." My voice trailed away. The world as I had known it was now shaky and uncertain.

"Well, I don't, not very often. Then my mother phones and asks me to come and do something for her - help with canning, or picking blueberries or - and there he is again! Sneaking in after everyone's in bed!" She crumpled in my arms, whimpering.

"Ask you mother to get a lock for your door," I suggested in sudden hope.

"I've told you, she won't listen! It's as if she knows, and doesn't want to hear it." This idea brought Hammond upright. "That's it!" she declared, wiping her eyes with her soaked handkerchief. "She knows! Next time I go home I'm going to make her listen!" Hammond squared her shoulders, resolve in every line of her body.

The next time Hammond went home on a night off I found an opportunity to ask her, "Did you tell your mother, Hammond?"

"I didn't try. What would she do? If she knew that I knew that she knew -" she laughed shakily - "she'd have to leave him. And what would she do? Where would she go?" In silence we contemplated the fate of an untrained housewife in the depths of the Depression.

"Does he still...?" I chanced the question. I could offer her a home with my parents.

"Not any more!" Hammond was triumphant. "I put a chain-lock on my door."

"Good for you! Let's go to the Tuck Shoppe and treat ourselves by way of celebration." I linked my arm with hers. The world had steadied again.

We breathed a sigh of relief when exams were finished. "No

lectures until January!" Gladwin was ecstatic. "Say, the new rosters are up and we're both on days. I'm going to ward H3. You're on H4, did you know?" Another top floor ward! What awaited me there?

Christmas Eve arrived, and both Dawson and I had to work. "Your first Christmas away from home?" Dawson inquired when we settled down at the table and the dormitory lights were out. "Your expression reminds me of my first Christmas here, and I had to work. I was on F3 days, and when all the patients were having their dinner in the dining room, my face must have looked as downcast as yours does now. The Charge came up to me and said, 'You can stop feeling sorry for yourself. You can go home, even if not on Christmas Day. These women can't, so get busy and don't let them see you with a sad face. They're the ones to feel sorry for.' It worked. You're off in a couple of nights, aren't you?"

That good advice worked for me too. Not only could the inmates not go home, many of them had no home to go to. Most never had a visitor. They were completely abandoned by their families.

Visitors were more frequent during Christmas week, though, and one of them caused the day and night staff on F3 a great deal of worry and trouble. Two days after Boxing Day the count was out by one patient, and the day staff could not leave until the missing woman was found. "Dead or alive," I immediately thought, and visions of possible means of suicide flashed through my mind. Everyone looked as worried as I felt.

McBride was in charge. "Dawson and I will redo the count," she stated, "and I want two of you with us, one in each dayroom." She named two of the day staff. "Start by clearing the washroom," she ordered, and they went off to their assigned task. Two more were sent to make a thorough check of the dormitory rooms. "Look under and behind every bed," they were told. "Check the dormitory washroom first. Vernon, you and Lehman go into every room along the entry corridor. I know they're all locked but anything is possible."

As we progressed along the corridor my expectations of finding a hanging body in the utility room, cut wrists in the kitchen, or a victim of poison in the dispensary were proved false, to my great relief. The linen room and clothes room were checked carefully; nobody was hiding there. "There's only the visitors' room left," said Vernon, "She can't have been left in there, but we'd better look anyway."

Vernon unlocked the door and we were faced by a blustering, obviously guilty man who launched an angry tirade against us. The woman we were searching for stood submissively, hands folded in front of her and head bowed. Visiting hours were over at four o'clock, and staff and patients had been past this room many times since then.

"What do you mean locking the door on me when I'm visiting my wife!" We recognized the falsity immediately; the door was never locked when the room was in use, but we were given no chance to speak. "I've been waiting two hours for someone to let me out. I've missed my supper, and my wife hasn't had hers. Heads are going to roll over this, you can be sure of that." Vernon was taking him out to the elevator as he kept raving, his face red – with rage or guilt? – and his voice loud and abusive.

Meanwhile I lost no time in taking the woman to the dayroom, and my explanation was met by mixed astonishment, barely suppressed laughter, and then a determination to find the culprits, the nurses who hadn't detected a missing person hours earlier.

"Who made the supper counts?" McBride's eyes swept her staff, and she quickly picked out the senior nurses looking very uncomfortable, with everyone's eyes on them. "Alright, you've been kept an extra half hour or more, but so has everyone else, and they know who is at fault. I don't have to remind you how important the count is, every time it is made. You counted into supper and back to the ward. Two counts were out. Don't let it happen again."

Dawson and I were left to begin the bedtime routine. "Three more nights to go, and this happens!" Dawson exclaimed. She broke into laughter. "I wish I'd been there to see his face. And he had the nerve to say he couldn't have banged on the door when he heard people passing by! It proves what they say, attack is the best defense! Wasn't he brazen, though!"

Our last three nights were uneventful. I would now discover whether ward H4 was as bad as its reputation alleged it to be.

CHAPTER NINE

There were two familiar faces on ward H4. "Hardy!" I exclaimed, as I joined the nurses lining up behind Miss Robertson the first morning. "Am I ever glad to see you here! You're the only one I know on this staff."

"They're a good crew," Hardy said. She looked sideways at me. "What do you suppose we did to be rewarded with a top floor ward again?" We walked over to work together.

"Isn't H4 the violent ward?" I asked. "I saw them in the dining room when we were on F4. They didn't look as messy and sluggish as ours. Miss Robertson looks pleasant." The Charge Nurse was pretty, though plumper than she probably wanted to be. Her cheeks had been carefully rouged and powdered, and a cupid's bow outlined her lips. Curly brown hair and friendly grey eyes completed an attractive appearance.

"Who is the Supervisor on H4?" I inquired idly. "Is she easy to work with?" Not that the staff saw much of the supervisors on the wards. Orders were relayed through or left entirely to the Charge.

"Miss Steele is nice but she has her own problems. You don't have to worry about her. There's no Skyler on this ward, either."

That was a relief. I was assigned to the dayroom with Clinton, a senior, after breakfast. Clinton was diminutive, more so even than Dawson, and I wondered at these illogical choices for psychiatric nurses. Then I was reminded of Miss Hicks, who held the highest position in the training school, and was herself a tiny person. My ideas of our vulnerability amongst violent patients would be tested on this ward.

The other familiar face was a patient. "Isn't that Queen Victoria?" I asked Clinton, as I spotted the regal figure seated in the dayroom, the same position she had commandeered on the ward two floors below. She wore the same outdated black clothes, the skirt spread around her to sweep the floor, and the assumed majestic air of the queen of England.

"Yes, that's Queenie," Clinton nodded.

"How did she get moved up here? She looks the same as she did on the other ward."

"Just watch her when Dr. Ryan makes rounds," Clinton advised. "She belongs up here all right. Apparently the H2 staff decided to make her take a much-needed bath and all hell broke loose! They didn't back down but they had to call for 'Help on H2!', an unheard-of happening. It took eight nurses to handle her, and I'll bet they had a time. She had to wear a ward dress while her clothes were sent to the laundry and that was when she acted up so much they transferred her up here, in a strait-jacket, straight to ward J. She didn't calm down until she got her own clothes again. Given the riot she raised and her temper, she was sent here instead of back to H2. There's a larger staff on here. She still goes wild every time Dr. Ryan appears. She has the notion he ordered a bath for her. It's an obsession. She calls him every name in the book."

Nearing the end of our first year of lectures, I could now match the behavior of patients to the categories of mental illness we had been studying. Queenie had grandiose delusions, and suffered persecutory beliefs. The facial distortions, tics, body jerks, and the withdrawal to another world of their own creation were no different than on other wards, but the H4 women were capable of violent reactions. There was an explosive quality on H4 such as that exhibited by Queenie when Dr. Ryan appeared.

"There he is, the double-dealing four-flusher! Nobody orders a bath for Queen Victoria! Don't come near me, you lying bastard! I'll have you hung, drawn and quartered. You're not a doctor, in your trumped-up white coat! You're a devil from hell and I hope you go there and fry your balls off!"

Dr. Ryan seemed unperturbed and Miss Hicks and Miss Marlatt disregarded the invective with their usual composure. I had my first look at Miss Steele, the ward supervisor. She, too, ignored Queenie's outburst. The problem Hardy had hinted at was her figure, I learned.

Overweight was Miss Steele's ruling concern.

"Stuffs herself, she does," Carmack said scornfully. Carmack was the senior nurse on the ward, next to Robertson, and she did not hesitate to discuss Miss Steele's problem the first time I was assigned to work with her.

Carmack herself was a big woman. In her 40s, she could best be described as robust and buxom. She carried her weight well, moving calmly and deliberately, and she spoke in the same way. Her Scottish accent, her age and her undoubted nursing expertise were signs of previous hospital experience, which she told me had been in a hospital in Scotland. She gave the impression of putting up with her present position but not liking it.

Carmack ate in the senior dining room, and there she heard about the means Miss Steele used to attempt to control her weight, while at the same time indulging herself in the rich foods she loved so much.

"Cutting down on food isn't in her book," Carmack scoffed. "Miss Steele thinks she can eat all she wants if she gets rid of it as soon as possible. Can you imagine sticking your finger down your throat after meals to make yourself vomit? And taking an enema every night? And does it do any good? Nossiree. She never loses a pound. Huh!"

Assisting another member of the staff in an unusual procedure proved to be an interesting experience. Robertson gave me instructions. "Lehman, I want you to go with Armstrong. She's taking Mrs. Whitt to our kitchen for her tube-feeding. Pay attention so you'll know how to do it." Miss Robertson's throaty voice always intrigued me. She sounded like Tallulah Bankhead, the movie star.

Armstrong, a senior nurse who reminded me of Richmond on my first ward, seated Mrs. Whitt in a chair, and to my amazement the patient opened her mouth to allow a rubber tube to be slipped down her throat. "Notice that the tube is marked to show how far you insert it," Armstrong said. She then started pouring a solution from a pitcher slowly into the funnel at the end of the tube. Mrs. Whitt sat quietly, not even gagging at a procedure that most people would find to be suffocating and painful.

"How long has she been fed like this?" I asked.

"Ever since she was admitted," Armstrong said. "About 18 months, she persists in an unshakable determination not to eat or drink." Mrs. Whitt showed no distress at her case being discussed. "She has to go to the dining room with the rest of the ward, as we can't leave her alone here, yet seeing everyone else eat doesn't seem to bother her. Every once in awhile we try to spoon-feed her but she refuses to take it."

"What's in the pitcher?" I asked. "Do you make it up?"

"No, it's mixed by the dietitian, and it must be nourishing as her weight doesn't change. The doctors are quite interested to see how long she can stay healthy without any solids."

When the pitcher was empty Armstrong withdrew the tube and I helped to clean the equipment. We returned the docile and apparently satisfied woman to the dayroom.

The dayrooms on H4 were decidedly noisy, more so than any other ward I had been on. Besides the quarreling and squabbling amongst volatile women, there were the moans and wails and cries of disturbed souls. Harrowing phrases were repeated endlessly throughout the day.

"My heart has turned upside down!" The jittery speaker wrung her hands in total despair, making an agitated circuit of the dayroom.

"An evil force has stolen my brain from me! I'm doomed!" A tormented woman rocked back and forth, her head between her hands.

Another woman was holding one arm up in front of her, stroking it, studying it, feeling it all over. "My arm is dead. I can't feel my arm. This is not my arm. Who took my arm, and left me this dead one?"

"My brain is melting. I can't think. I can't remember anything. I might as well be dead!" The agony expressed was very real and could not be appeased. We tried to ignore what could not be helped.

We also ignored the curses and obscenities directed at the demons that possessed their minds. Occasionally the nurses were blasted with vitriolic intensity, and sometimes we were spit at in demonic fury. "I can take anything but spitting," Carmack declared. "Then I do have to hang on to my temper."

A beautiful olive-skinned woman paced the floor, raising her arms to shake her fists at intervals, and chanting in a foreign tongue.

There was an air of volcanic passion about her.

"Murdered her husband, that one did," Carmack commented dryly. "Probably had good reason to. She doesn't bother anyone as long as she's left alone. It's too bad we can't understand what she's saying."

"What about that one sitting by the window, with blood oozing out of a gouge on her forehead?" I wondered if she had been scratched by another patient. But it was more of a gash than a scratch.

"That woman has tic douloureux," Carmack said, with pity in her voice. "It's a nerve disorder. She feels such pain along the course of the nerve that she scratches to 'let it out.' It's bad this afternoon. I'll go and tell Miss Steele and she'll step up her medication. Dr. Ryan leaves a standing order for her."

The definition of 'tic douloureux' in my medical dictionary was 'An acutely painful neuralgia of the face with paroxysmal muscular twitchings.' It would not be surprising if such physical misery led to mental upsets, such as the wish to take her own life. Or a lashing-out at the people around her.

There were withdrawn patients on H4, too. The extreme phase of catatonia, when the muscles become rigid, was rare, and because it alternated with phases of excitement, was not a permanent condition. We did have to feed the catatonic patient, though, and food was accepted and swallowed. Our tube-fed woman, Mrs. Whitt, was not catatonic. In all respects except her obdurate refusal to eat, Mrs. Whitt was no different than any withdrawn patient.

Sometimes the nurses could see turbulence building up and sometimes an eruption occurred without warning. Early in my training I had been instructed in the arm hold that we were to use in controlling a patient. We were to grab the patient's right wrist with our right hand and twist that arm behind her back, which is not painful unless the arm is raised too far upward. The nurse's left arm is wrapped around the patient's neck, and kept under the chin to prevent her from wriggling out of the hold. As the nurse is behind the patient she can propel her forward in ordinary cases of disobedience or intractability. We had recourse to the call for 'help on H4' when the patient was truly wild and several nurses were needed to quell the violent woman.

As on ward F4, there were half a dozen cells or single rooms on H4, used for short term isolation. There were no padded cells in the building, as sedatives were used to protect the patient from herself.

An unusual alliance between two patients on H4 made the staff uneasy. We felt fairly secure in our ability to handle one patient; but nobody relished the thought of two women ganging up against us. The two women were both named Campbell, and were known as 'Big Campbell,' nearly six feet tall and of massive build, and 'Little Campbell,' who was so named only to differentiate between the two. Little Campbell was of average height, but with powerful shoulders and an aggressive, swaggering walk. They were a formidable pair.

"I hope those two cool off soon," Carmack said, as we watched their martial progress along the corridor on the way to the dining room. Side by side, they marched in step with a belligerence that boded ill for anyone in their way.

"I'd swear they're planning something, the way they whisper together and look at us," said Hardy, looking worried. Events proved her to be correct.

The conspirators chose their time well. The Supervisor was off the ward for her two-hour dinner break, Robertson had taken early dinner herself, so there was no one in the office to make a quick phone call for help. Armstrong and Carmack were also off the ward, sent directly to dinner from the patients' dining room. That left Clinton, not more than an inch over five feet tall, easy-going Hardy and myself in charge of the patients.

Clinton said, "I see my dormitory workers by the porch in the second dayroom. I want to explain the extra work to be done this afternoon." And she scooted off. Hardy and I continued to talk idly.

"Do you live nearby," I asked, "so you can get home on your days off?"

"I live on a farm a mile past the Red Bridge. How about you?"

"I can take the bus into town and get the early bus back for lectures, but lots of times I stay in the Home. It's such a treat to stay in bed when the wake-up bell goes..."

"Miss Hardy! Miss Lehman! Come quick! The Campbells are after Miss Clinton's keys!" A patient was calling us as she ran in from the other room.

We raced into the second dayroom to see a struggle going on in the far corner. Clinton was barricaded behind an easy chair, tugging back on her key-strap which was attached securely to the belt around her waist. Little Campbell had the key in her hand, and several women were trying to loosen her hold on it. Big Campbell was pushing the women away with her powerful arms, but they came swarming back.

"I'll get on the phone," Hardy said as soon as she saw that Clinton was besieged but not hurt. She ran back to the office.

Big Campbell was effectively stopped from helping her partner by a heavy patient who had jumped onto her back and had a strangle hold around her neck, while the other women kept close in front of her. I waded into the fight that was going on with Little Campbell, and the patients who had so valiantly been helping gave way to the stream of nurses who started arriving. By their sheer numbers the nurses soon regained control.

"You must have asked for lots of help," I said to Hardy when we were walking back from the dormitory where the two Campbells had been put into separate rooms to cool off. Robertson and the other two from our staff had returned from their dinner, and the extra nurses had gone back to their wards.

"I said there were two on the rampage, It's a good thing you didn't get hurt, Clinton. How did you get behind the chair?"

"Mrs. Barwick saw them advancing on me and yelled, 'The Campbells are after you!' and I was over that chair before I had time to think. Maudie jumped on Big Campbell's back and kept her out of it. It's a good thing my workers were with me. That's one thing those two hadn't figured on, I guess. Little Campbell got at my keys as I was going over the chair but the women kept her from me, bless them. I hope none of them are hurt."

"I'll check them, Clinton," Robertson said. "You three go off for your dinner now. You'll be late. Take the full three-quarters of an hour anyway. We'll have to move one of the Campbells off the ward, but which one?"

In a few days Little Campbell was allowed back into the dayroom and Big Campbell was moved to ward H3. I asked Gladwin how she fitted in there.

"No trouble so far," was the answer. "In fact she looks quite deflated without Little Campbell who was the more aggressive one. I'm sure glad they didn't go after us on nights. I didn't trust those two at all."

"You know, what I find so different from what I expected in this place is the friendliness of so many of the women, when they're not in a manic phase. And with the number who are wrapped up in themselves and their own troubles, that leaves very few who might attack a nurse, even on the top floor." I was becoming almost too complacent as a psychiatric nurse.

"We haven't been on ward J yet," Gladwin warned. "They have to be taken out of the siderooms for the toilet and showers. I wouldn't even want to be on nights there."

"Well, I think I've had my share of the worst wards already, but you know, they're not as bad as people on the outside may think."

One afternoon, Hardy and I were given the pleasant task of taking some women to a patients' dance in the Male Chronic Building.

"You haven't been to a dance here, Lehman? You'll enjoy it," Robertson said, smiling. "You'll meet some attendants and you can dance, too. You might get asked by a male patient and you can't refuse, but they're OK if they're at the dance. You should have a good time."

Our patients were waiting for us in the rotunda, and we set off for the far building. Mrs. Barwick was among them. "It's my only chance to play the piano," she said.

One of the dayrooms in the Male Chronic Building had the furniture moved to the side and the carpets rolled up, leaving a beautiful hardwood floor for the dancing. Robertson was right; I did enjoy myself and the men and women certainly had a good time. There were some good dancers among them.

Mrs. Barwick moved to the piano and played waltzes and fox trots for an hour and a half, all without music in front of her. While I was on H4 though, she was brought back from one of the dances sobbing uncontrollably and profoundly agitated.

"She was playing just fine at first," Carmack told us. "Then she started speeding it up and pounding the keys like mad, and we had to practically lift her off the piano stool. She came back without any trouble, just crying so hard she couldn't see where she was going.

Must have been the music that upset her."

Mrs. Barwick was sedated and put to bed for the rest of the day and returned to the dayroom the next day, subdued but in a state of agitation. She muttered continually, pacing about and looking out the window at the parking lot in front of the building.

"Her husband was here the other day to visit her," Clinton remembered. "She's always upset after his visits. It's a good thing he doesn't come very often."

"Mrs. Barwick plays a good hand of bridge," Carmack said. "We've nothing to do for the next while. There's three of us here now. You can play, can't you, Lehman? Come on, you don't have to be an expert and it might keep her mind off her worries." We played at one of the dayroom tables.

Mrs. Barwick joined us willingly but was the oddest player I could have imagined. Her muttering never ceased, yet she kept track of the bids and played the cards as well as anyone around the table.

"Sweet-talking me while his lady-love waits in the car for him to get my money. One spade. I've seen her out there. He doesn't bother to visit until the money runs out---three diamonds---but when he wants a cheque signed or bonds turned over to him it's 'Mollie, love' and 'Sweetheart' and kissing and cooing. Four spades." And she proceeded to make her bid, mumbling continually while she took in the tricks.

"I think she's got something to complain about," Clinton said when the game was over and Mrs. Barwick had returned to her post at the window. "I've seen a woman waiting out there in the car he got into after his visit."

One of our patients had developed a strong body odor that we couldn't trace to its source. She showered regularly and had clean clothes. The hospital dentist checked her mouth and her teeth. They were healthy. The rotten smell persisted, and the other women hated to be near her, especially in the dining room.

"Bring Miss Darby to the dispensary, Lehman," Robertson told me one day. "Dr. Campbell is going to examine her. You can stay to take her back to the dayroom afterward."

Robertson and Miss Steele were ready when I brought the woman in. We had her undressed and lying on an examining table when Dr. Campbell arrived, accompanied by Miss Hicks and Miss Marlatt. Miss Darby was covered by a sheet and her heels were in stirrups.

The doctor made a complete check of her body and then went to the foot of the table to make a vaginal examination. "There's something in here! Forceps, please," he said. To the amazement of the onlookers, he drew out a stinky gold watch, turned greeny black and covered with slime. The smell, bad before was overpowering. Miss Marlatt had a handkerchief to her nose.

"Wait, there's something else," Dr. Campbell exclaimed. This time he placed a heart-shaped locket beside the watch on the tray. We watched in fascination as he found a badly-decomposed article. "I think this was a leather change purse," he said - followed by two slimy rings, a small souvenir spoon, and a lipstick case. All were discolored and covered with mucous. The stench was awful.

"A vinegar douche now, Miss Steele," the doctor said, "and repeat until the vagina is clean. Then we'll see if there are any more treasures in there." His eyes were twinkling as he went over to the sink to remove his rubber gloves and scrub his hands.

"Shall I wrap these up and get rid of them?" Robertson asked, eyeing the filthy objects, her nose wrinkled.

"Oh, I think we'll keep them," Dr. Campbell said. "The other doctors will want to see them. but do wash them off as well as you can, and use a disinfectant. We don't need that smell." Miss Hicks had opened the window section that was on hinges, and stayed by it for fresh air. Everyone wore a look of bemusement mixed with suppressed laughter.

My account of the vaginal cache was received with disbelief and incredulous amusement in the Home that night. "You're kidding, Lehman! Those things wouldn't stay up there while she walked around all the time! A watch? I don't believe you!"

"Wouldn't her husband get a surprise if she'd been married!" was Dunbar's first thought.

"Well! Now we know where to stash our valuables!" Ferrier remarked.

"I don't think so," was Oliver's quiet rejoinder. To that I heartily agreed.

CHAPTER TEN

Marshall burst into our room the first day of February. "Hey, I'm off nights at last!" We had just come off duty. "And what, may I ask, have you two been up to these long winter evenings?"

"The same old thing, work and lectures," I said, rubbing my feet after kicking off my duty shoes.

"Well, let's get going! Have you ever gone over to the Boys' Industrial School?"

Gladwin and I looked at one another. "Why should we go there?" I wondered aloud. The yellow buildings for boys in trouble with the law were further along the hillside from the mental hospital.

"We're allowed to use the gymnasium one night a week, and tonight's the night. There are no lectures so why don't we go. There are also badminton courts with racquets and shuttlecocks. You've never played? It's easy; you'll soon get on to it. There's a swimming pool too..."

"A pool the bad boys use?" said Gladwin, wrinkling her nose. "Not for me! It'll be full of pee. But I'd like to play badminton. You'll go, Lehman? Give us ten minutes to change, Marshall."

"I have to change too, and I'll see if I can round up a couple more." Marsahll was out the door as she spoke.

We had walked along the low stone wall that fronted the grounds of the institution and were starting up the winding driveway that led to the buildings. "I feel like I'm trespassing," I said with a shiver.

"It's knowing there's eyes at every window watching us," Marshall laughed. "But, I've never seen any boys outside the buildings. Yet they must be out sometimes, I guess when we're at work. D'you suppose the guards have guns?" It was a sobering thought.

The gloomy gymnasium was stuffy and smelled of sweat. "Smells of dirty feet," Langley sniffed and coughed. "Why do boys' feet smell more than girls'?"

"Because they wear sneakers all day, I guess," Gladwin said. We were changing into our running shoes. We swatted the shuttlecocks across the net with more enthusiasm than skill for the next hour.

"You'll be champions by the time the evenings are lighter and we'll be going for walks again," Marshall predicted. "How about the Saturday night dance? Are you game to go?"

"Not me," said Gladwin firmly. "Saturday night is my regular date with Don."

"I'm for it," Langley said simultaneously with my "Sure thing! Who else is going?"

"Hammond would like to come. I've already spoken to her about it. That's four of us. Enough for Bob's old jalopy. But he can't take us there; he'll bring us home. He has to help his father milk the cows and by the time he gets cleaned up we'd be late and miss some of the dancing if we waited for him to pick us up. It's not far to walk, about a mile. Oh, be sure to ask Miss Hicks for a one o'clock leave. Just tell her you're going to the old-time dance. She approves of that."

Saturday evening saw us starting out in the cold winter air, walking briskly across the Red Bridge toward Port Coquitlam. We carried shoes for dancing and had our extra late leaves in the pockets of our heavy coats. "Are we going to the Aggie Hall?" I asked.

"No, there's a hall closer than that. It's the ballroom of a big old building that was supposed to be a hotel, though why anyone would build a hotel so far out of town beats me. Ask some of the local boys about it. They'd know more than I do."

We turned off Shaughnessy Street, which became the main street of the town farther along, and passed the school grounds. Here the houses became scarce and the trees hadn't been cleared from most of the lots.

It was a shock to come upon a large white building here. Wings stretched back on each side of the central portion which faced the road. Heavy carved double doors led into what had undoubtedly been the lobby. It was bare except for the beautifully carved reception desk where we paid our 25 cents. A lively square dance tune was struck up in the large room to our left. Hurriedly changing into our lighter shoes, we were swept into the squares that were forming for the first dance. A fiddler and a piano player provided the music and a grizzled man in a western shirt and cowboy hat called the movements. "First couple up to the right...Birdie fly in and hawkie fly out...Over and under, under and over..." It was fun. Everyone was dancing.

During the break for refreshments I asked the questions posed by this white elephant of a building. I had noted the ceiling decorations, the plaster broken and darkened after so many years, but definitely ostentatious in its concept. "What on earth is a hotel doing in the middle of nowhere, anyway? Was it ever used as a hotel?"

Tim and Walter looked at one another. "To tell you the truth I never thought about it," Walter said lightheartedly. "It was always here, and a religious group were in it until about five years ago. I guess I figured they'd built it."

"No, it's a hotel right enough," Tim said. "I've heard it was built when the railway was coming this way, and people thought that Port Coquitlam was to be the terminus."

"But who would put their money into a hotel so far from the railway line?" I asked. "It must be at least half-a-mile away. I'll bet it was meant for something like a hospital!"

"No, let me tell you what I've heard," Tim said. "Come along and look at the rooms and the set-up. The whole thing sounds impossible, all right, but how else do you explain it? Anyone else want to come?"

Hammond and Walter went with us across the lobby, which also had rosettes worked into the plastered ceiling. There was a wide staircase rising to the second floor. Tim passed this and we entered a corridor on the right.

"There aren't any lights connected in this part of the building," Tim said, lighting a match and holding it up. "You can see this hall goes down the length of this wing---ouch!" He threw the match on the floor and stepped on it, then lit another. We all stopped in the dim light from the lobby, not wanting to go on into the darkness.

Tim was saying, "There's rooms on each side, and both wings upstairs have rooms each side of the center hall."

"Sounds like you've been through it in daylight." I had seen enough to convince me and we turned back. "You said you'd heard who built it and why. Come on, why don't you tell us all about it."

"Well I don't know his name, or even where he lived, but it was financed by someone who didn't live here, that's for sure. Sit on the steps here and I'll tell you the way I heard it."

It was a fascinating story, and my imagination filled in the details Tim didn't provide in his brief outline before the dancing resumed. Someone back east, with money to invest, saw the opportunities presented by the railway being built across the country, and determined to put his money into a hotel at the end of the line. Someone at this end, either unscrupulous or badly misinformed, bought lots for him at the inflated prices that prevailed with the promise of Port Coquitlam being the terminus, and built this imposing hotel.

Certainly it was built in a grand manner. The carved front doors and reception desk and the ballroom where we were dancing bespoke of grand expectations. The opening of this part of the country to entrepreneurs assured the investor of good business for his hotel at the end of the railway line.

"When he finally came out himself, probably on the first train to come through, he had to hire a rig to drive him out here. When he saw how isolated it was, more so 50 years ago than now, he shot himself." Tim spoke matter-of-factly but there was mischief in his eyes.

"Shot himself!" Hammond and I jumped up. The music was starting in the other room. "Where?" We looked around us, as if expecting to see a dead body with a smoking pistol in its hand.

"Probably right where you're standing," Walter chuckled. "Come on, the dancing's starting. That was a long time ago."

We learned something of what it was like to be a young man in the 30s from talking to them at the dances. There were absolutely no prospects for employment of any kind, no chance of establishing themselves or hopes of being able to support a family. Hope was something that died hard, yet the reality was all around them, starting with their own parents' struggle to get the necessities of life.

Tim, who seemed so easy-going on first acquaintance, revealed a deep-seated bitterness as we got to know him. He had a stocky frame and squashed-in features, hardly good-looking, but he was honest, and very serious about 'getting ahead.'

He was studying the soles of his shoes during the refreshment break one night. "They're getting so thin I can't walk on gravel," he said. "If I didn't wear work boots here and change into these when I get here I'd soon be dancing in the work boots. And I guess I step on enough toes as it is. I sure wish I could get a steady job."

"What have you been doing, Tim?" I asked sympathetically.

My tone must have unleashed months of held-in anger. "Damn well nothing, that's what! The few dollars I made fruit picking won't stretch any farther. I hate having to ask my father for a quarter to go to a movie or to pay for the dance. I know I earn it helping on the farm but I know damn well the milk check barely buys what my parents need. It doesn't help my self-respect to have to live off them. I'm 18. It's time I was able to support myself." He brooded for a moment.

"My mom doesn't want me to go but I'm going east. There must be work in Ontario with all the factories and industries there. If I could just be at the right place when a job opens up..."

"How will you get there, Tim? You won't hop a freight, will you?" But I knew from his obdurate expression that he would. There was no other way, when you had no money.

Young men were going east looking for work, and men from the east and from the prairies were coming west to British Columbia, and they all rode in or on top of freight cars. Vancouver was a mecca for the homeless in the winter. The prospects of getting work were no better than anywhere else but at least the days of tramping the streets and the nights of rolling up in a blanket in whatever shelter they could find - under a bridge, in a shed or an empty warehouse - would be less bitterly cold than in the place they came from.

How did they eat? Soup kitchens were in operation all across Canada in the 30s, some of them set up in the bad times a decade earlier, but now feeding much greater numbers than ever before. I remembered homeless men when I was growing up on the farm. They were professional hoboes. It was a way of life.

Our dog would start barking long before the ragged man appeared. Mother made up thick sandwiches which she passed out to him to eat on the step, or in the shelter of the porch in bad weather. Even the dog kept his distance from the unwashed and unkempt men.

Sometimes, when the man had eaten, he picked up the axe that rested on the chopping block by the pile of wood, and cut up some wood as pay for his food. More often he plodded wearily on his way to nowhere. Another farm, another meal. Another day.

Tim would be among a different company. The men and boys who hopped the freight cars slept and ate in 'jungles' along the railway line. There was a jungle in Kamloops, and one in Chilliwack. Port Moody harbored a jungle, as did New Westminster, and there was one under the Georgia Viaduct in Vancouver. Vagrants gathered there, building a fire for warmth and to cook the food they had begged or stolen. There they found companionship in their wretchedness.

The brick factory at Kilgard, a few miles out of Abbotsford, had its share of hoboes, drawn by the heat of the kilns. The women in the company town were accustomed to an organized form of begging. A man would ask for one egg at one door, a second one at the next house. Someone else was asking for slices of bread, and maybe a chicken would be appropriated. Anyone dropping into their camp that night shared in a good meal.

But the unemployed of the 20s following the return of the servicemen from the war was as nothing to the glut of the 30s, when countless hopeless men wandered the country looking for non-existent work.

Some of the other fellows we danced with had tried the freight car method of travelling. Stan, a tall thin young man was back home after making a few dollars during harvest on the prairies. He spoke resentfully of the treatment by the railway guards who were hired to try to keep the men off the trains.

"How else were we to travel?" he asked. "Who has the money to buy a ticket?"

He told of his buddy's bad luck, jumping off the train when it slowed down for a station.

"We'd get off before it stopped, walk through the town to avoid the guards and catch that one or the next one on the other side before it got up too much speed. My buddy didn't see the culvert that ran under the tracks and he landed right on the darn thing. Broke his leg, and skinned it plenty too. Thank God for the Red Cross. They looked after him. Any time I get any extra money it's going to the Red Cross. They have a heart."

Stan was especially bitter about railway guards - the 'bulls', he called them. "They caught me in Kamloops - what was I doing wrong? The trains are on the tracks anyway - what harm were we doing? Those ..." his language became profane, ending with, "bloody bulls threw me in jail. In jail! For nothing more than what tons of other guys are doing every day, riding the freights. So now I have a criminal record." He glowered. There was nothing I could say.

The boys we danced with had tried everything. Chester had been mining in Alberta, until the constant darkness below ground made him so claustrophobic he had to quit. "I haven't got the coal grime out of my hands yet," he said, showing us blackened nails. "But say, I learned something about mules. Do you know there's mules that are kept underground and they never see daylight? Boy are they smart! They pull the loaded coal cars, you see, and I don't know how they do it but they won't pull one car over the regular load. I swear they can count. I've seen the guys try to distract them while one fellow is coupling an extra car way back at the end of the train, and that mule won't move. Won't even attempt to pull. Just stands there, stubborn as - a mule! He has to have counted the cars that were hitched. Take one off, and that mule ups and away." He shook his head. "I'll never understand it."

The fellows talked about the chances of work. "Can't get hop picking on Sumas Prairie, even. The Indians have that all sewed up. There's three interurban cars leave New Westminster every morning just for hop pickers, and they're mostly Indians."

Berry picking didn't pay much, and women and kids did most of it. Tobacco was being grown near Yarrow but the young men nearby got the work in the fields while the tobacco and hops were being planted and cultivated, then there was a short season of tobacco picking. Fruit picking in the Okanagan was good for a few dollars, and there was work in the packing plants in Penticton and

Kamloops. "If you can get there ahead of everyone else," one fellow said dryly.

"I wouldn't even mind working at Essondale," one young man said. "Especially at Colony Farm. But someone's brother or cousin gets any job that comes vacant."

"What about the relief camps?" Walter asked. "The government in Ottawa is setting them up now. Has anyone been in the ones B.C. started last year?"

"Yeah, that's something else," Chester said. "Some are O.K. but some of those bosses think they have you in the army. And I guess they have, in a way. Do as they say or get out. A friend of mine was in one in some godforsaken place up country. It's just a scheme to get men off the streets of Vancouver anyway. He said the bosses didn't care so the men took their time - it was all make-work stuff, nothing useful. They'd sit around by the road they were supposed to be making, from nowhere to nowhere, and play cards or tell jokes or whatever. Pretty dull life. And they got paid 20 cents a day! A dollar a week! Nothing to do and nowhere to go in the evenings. The 20 cents bothered some of them more than if they'd been given nothing but board and a place to sleep. They said it was an insult. Depends on how you look at it, I guess."

We flirted mildly with our partners but we knew there was no future in our friendships, until the job situation improved. None of us knew it wouldn't until the next war started in 1939, and even then war plants weren't providing work for a few years after that. Many of the young people joined the army, not because they wanted to fight, but to get clothed and fed, and most important, paid.

The men had it hard in the Depression, but women had a hard time, too. Somehow the family had to be fed. Farm women made butter and sold it, along with eggs from chickens that were their responsibility to keep. They took worn shirt collars off, picking out the stitches carefully, turned the good side out and sewed the collars back on. A sewing machine was a necessity. Mothers made clothes for their children from worn-out suits and dresses of their own. Children's clothing, including shoes, were passed down from the oldest to the youngest with much patching along the way.

Household goods wore out too. Clotheslines held ragged towels and sheets sewn down the middle. Everyone knew that when a sheet was worn thin, you could rip it down the middle and sew the sides together. Hem the new sides, carefully, for the material was worn thin, and the sheet was good for another year. When the sheet finally wore through again, there was enough material at the top and bottom to make pillow slips.

Women canned fruits and vegetables and meat, when an animal was butchered. They didn't have refrigeration to make it easy to keep the meat. They baked bread and if the wood was green and wet they dried enough of it in the oven to keep the fire going. On the farm, the men usually went into the woods to cut down trees and get in a supply of wood. There wasn't much time to worry about hard times. Most farms had a radio and everybody listened to The Happy Gang, Ma Perkins, Jack Benny and all the other wonderful radio programs of the 30s. The hard times would come to an end some day.

There was no future in sexual intimacy, for who could afford to get married? The very real possibility of pregnancy was a strong deterrent. We knew that some girls 'went all the way', for we saw the hurried marriage and the drudgery of life without money, or the plight of the girl who was left to bear the burden alone.

So we enjoyed the dances, and baseball games in a farm field, and rides in somebody's old jalopy, and believed that better times must be around the corner. They had to be!

For most of that spring I was going out with Hal, an Essondale attendant I had met at a patients' dance. Though Hal didn't dance, we liked each other and he had started calling at the Nurses' Home for me for walks in the evenings. It was Hal who told me the Home was known as the 'Chicken Coop.' I was faintly offended, but I could see the point. "It looks like one," he said hastily, when he saw my reaction. "That's all."

Hal was anxious to please, obviously a well-brought up young lad. He was stockily built, with the largest hands I have ever seen. I was not surprised when he told me he did some wrestling. I was amazed to learn he was also an artist.

Shyly he presented me with a gauzy handkerchief one night, the corners painted in delicate designs. "It's not perfect," he said, pointing out a little squiggle here and there. "It's my first attempt at a handkerchief, but I wanted to give you something pretty. I've only worked in oils, doing landscapes mostly."

"You didn't do this!" I exclaimed thoughtlessly, glancing at his ham-like hands.

"You don't believe me, huh?" he said, crushed. "Just like you don't believe I'm serious about getting married." Hal hadn't asked me to marry him. He just assumed we had a future together and I always refused to take him seriously . He didn't know how young I was and I couldn't tell him and risk the word getting around to Miss Hicks. I was certainly not ready to settle down to housework and family responsibilities.

By this time I knew Hal's father was dead and that he was the only son. One night he announced, "I'm taking you to meet my mother."

They lived in a small, neat house on the outskirts of Port Coquitlam, about a half hour walk from the hospital. Hal told me he lived at home, though there were attendants' quarters on the hill back of the Male Chronic Building. "I can help out at home this way," he said. "Cut the lawn and stuff like that. I do all the gardening, too." There was pride in his voice as he showed me his roses and flowers that were coming up from bulbs he had planted. Hal was a curious mix of strength and artistic bent, and I was increasingly attracted to him.

He opened the front door and called, "Mother?" The house was strangely quiet and rather gloomy with all the blinds drawn, though it was still light outside.

"In here, son." A quavering voice drew us into a darkened bedroom, and one small light showed that his mother was in bed. She looked at me coldly as Hal introduced us.

"You work in the asylum?" she asked, making it sound like a crime. Her unfriendly eyes didn't quite meet mine.

Puzzled, for her son worked there too, I answered, "I'm taking nurses' training there, yes." We were standing by her bedside, and the situation made me uncomfortable.

"Hmph!" she sniffed. "Nurses! Drinking beer, and smoking..."

"Mother," Hal said patiently. "Eva doesn't drink, or smoke." But his mother didn't want to hear that. She sniffed again, and put a handkerchief to her nose. I looked at Hal and turned to the door, knowing that nothing I could say would overcome her prejudice.

Hal started to leave with me but his mother detained him with a request that he plump up her pillows, then she needed a drink of water. I realized that she wanted me to know that her son was at her beck and call, and the absence of any sign of welcome told me she didn't want to share him with anyone.

"I didn't know your mother was an invalid," I said, "Was she expecting me?"

"I told her I was bringing you." Hal sounded puzzled. "She must have taken a bad turn or something like that."

As always, opposition roused my fighting instinct, and I began to count up Hal's good points. He was kind, and he was honest. He had a steady job. He was short, but not shorter than I was. He was not bad-looking. On the other hand, he didn't dance, and I loved dancing. Maybe I could teach him... Somehow wrestling and dancing didn't go together. And where would we live? I suspected his wages kept the home going, and his mother would never accept me. Nor I her!

Then Hal revealed his dream, which was absolutely contrary to the way I hoped to live.

"When we're married," he began, "we'll live on a ranch in the Cariboo country. In a log cabin. I've always wanted to build a log cabin. We'll have a cow and some chickens. And you'll get up in the mornings and light the fire..." Only someone who had never lived on a farm could be romantic and dreamy about it as Hal was at that moment. We were sitting on a bench in a secluded area of the hospital grounds, his arm around me, my head on his shoulder.

I sat up straight. "It's late," I said. "I have to be in. And Hal, I don't think we should see each other any more." Nothing he could say would change my mind. My aversion to farming was based on the years I grew up on one. The fact that I could so quickly decide not to see Hal again told me I hadn't been in love with him. I had been in love with love, and I liked the prestige of having a young man call upon me at the Nurses' Home.

When the doorbell was answered and a young man asked for one of the nurses, he was escorted into a visitors' room just inside the front door, always by whoever was closest for Miss Whitehorse ignored the bell and the phone. Then the girl's name was shouted, just as it was for a phone call, only this time the word "Visitor!" followed, and everyone knew she had a boyfriend. That satisfaction wouldn't be mine any more. I would miss Hal, too, but the conditions of my early years on the farm had been brought back vividly to me recently on a visit to Hardy's home. Farm conditions could be decent, or they could be primitive. And when they were primitive, it was a hard life. Especially for the women.

Hardy heard me saying I'd be staying in the Home on a day off because my parents were away. "I'm off too, Lehman," she said. "Why don't you come home with me? It's only a little more than a mile to walk." I knew Hardy lived on a farm on the Pitt River road.

So it was that we set out across the Red Bridge and on around the base of Mary Hill, dropping down into the flat lands that bordered the Pitt River. "Here we are," Hardy said, lifting the wire loop that fastened the gate, then closing it behind us.

I saw a log house at the end of a weed-choked path. Chickens and geese scratched in the yard. Some make-shift sheds and a log barn with an odorous manure pile stood not far from the back of the house. "You grew up on a farm, didn't you?" Hardy's eyes slid apologetically toward me.

Yes, I thought, but our farm was far different from this. My father took pride in his carpentry skills and he had built a large, two-storied house, finished in white clapboard. There were three bedrooms, a kitchen, dining room and living room. The pantry was lined with cupboards and was equipped with a sink, with hot and cold running water. Dad had laid the water pipes himself, after sinking a well in a stream above the house. A bathroom had been fitted into a corner of the back porch that ran the length of the house. It had a tub, a basin and a toilet. I barely remembered the outside toilet of my early years, with Eaton's catalogue used for toilet paper.

We had a telephone in the last few years, but still didn't have electricity. I had painful memories of the hours I spent churning butter - first with a dasher that was pumped up and down by hand in a large jar. Then we had a churn which made butter with paddles that were turned by a handle on the side. Lastly, I pumped a treadle on a barrel-type churn which swished back and forth, back and forth until the butter formed. The cream was often not cold enough, as we had no refrigeration.

Clothes were scrubbed on a washboard in the early years, a job guaranteed to skin the knuckles. Then a hand-operated machine appeared on our back porch, and I did my share of pushing and pulling the handle on the top of the wooden tub to turn it in a half-circle. My mother still boiled the clothes first in an oval copper washtub that fitted over the fire-box of the wood range.

And the entrance! Dad had constructed a stone fence that enclosed the lawn and flowers my mother kept, and curved it in to the driveway - a farm driveway, two ruts and grass between. The hip-roofed barn with cattle stalls below and a hay-loft above, was a good distance downhill from the house, and the obligatory manure pile was not discernible by sight or smell.

All of this was the result of their own hard work for the hillside farm was virgin land when they bought it. It had to be cleared of trees and stumps before buildings could go up.

All this went through my mind the evening we were going in to meet Hardy's folks. Farms differed, it is true, but all of them are seven-day-a-week operations, I knew. And farm prices had not been good in years.

Hardy's father, mother and eight-year-old brother sat around the oilcloth covered kitchen table in the hot, white light of a gas lamp hanging from a beam overhead. There was one big room for eating, sleeping, and sitting in the evenings.

"Here you are!" Mrs. Hardy was mending socks. "Just put your things on Willie's bed," and she gestured toward the dim recesses outside the light. Two double beds stood against a side and a back wall. "Sit here," she nodded toward a chair, and smiled at me.

Mr. Hardy and Wilbert sat on a bench behind the table, one with the newspaper the other with his homework in front of him. They nodded at me and resumed reading. Hardy stayed at the back of the room, folding and putting away clean clothes that had been brought in from the line and dumped on the bed. She and her mother exchanged news while they worked. A pig had been butchered, and the price of eggs had dropped again. Hardy's new assignment was OK.

I looked around this room where I would be sleeping and eating for tonight and tomorrow. If my father hadn't taken carpentry work while my mother kept the farm chores going, we might have been living in conditions like this. Our hillside land wasn't suitable for farming and dad was not a farmer, though he must have thought he could be at one time. In the good years before the crash, he had planted an orchard and put in the posts and wire for my mother's raspberry patch, and ground was broken for strawberries and potatoes and all kinds of vegetables, so there was food to eat.

City friends thought that's all there was to it. They drove out to see us and mother killed a chicken to feed them, and they went home with fruit and berries and vegetables in their cars. My mother did most of the weeding and cultivating and picking off suckers and pruning and whitewashing the trunks of the fruit trees. She cut out the dead raspberry canes and tied the new growth to the wires to withstand the winter winds, and hoed around the roots after dad drove the horse-drawn cultivator through the patch. She cleaned out the chicken coop - and she chopped the chicken heads off with an ax to feed our company, cleaned the insides out and plucked the feathers off, while everyone else talked and laughed inside. It was anything but an easy life, for a woman.

The big black wood-burning stove here was the same as the one in our farm kitchen. The fire-box was on the left and the oven was beside it under a polished black top surface. A warming oven rose up at the back and loomed over the stove, and a drying rack for clothes was suspended over it, raised and lowered by means of ropes and a pulley.

One of my chores on the farm had been to keep the wood-box filled, carrying in armloads of split wood to pile in the capacious box that was built in under the stairs in our house.

How well I remembered the sad-irons, exactly the same as the three that were on this stove, pushed out of the way at the back while not in use. On ironing day the fire had to be hot, and the irons were rotated over the heat by means of a snap-on handle. It took adroit handling of irons and feeding wood at just the right time, to be able to iron heavily starched dresses and shirts without burning holes in them, yet get them smooth with no wrinkles.

My mother tells the story of my 'helping hand' when I was three years old. She had made starch and left it to cool in a bowl on the stove while she went out on the porch and did the wash - this was before the sink and running water had been put in. The clothes had been boiled and the kettle emptied to make the starch, so she let the fire go out.

This busy little bee pulled a chair up to the stove which was only comfortably warm now, piled the breakfast dishes from the dishpan into the starch, and washed the dishes for Mummy. Mother came in to use the starch - disaster!

Wood stoves were used in the city as well as on farms. Then sawdust and oil, and even coal, became popular, until electricity with all its advantages came into use a decade later.

Where would Hardy and I wash up? A high kitchen cupboard near the stove was flanked by a shelf with a water bucket and a dishpan on it. A half-full slop pail stood on the floor below. There was a bench at the side door with a hand basin on it and a family towel hanging beside it. The kettle steaming on the stove would provide hot water.

Mr. Hardy lit a lantern and went out, the signal for Mrs. Hardy to fold the socks and make up a bed for Wilbert. He would sleep on two benches from around the table, placed side by side at the back, while we occupied his bed in the corner.

In turn we took the lantern and went out to the privy, Hardy going with me to show me the way. Thistles and uncut grass around the outhouse were perfect hiding places for creepy, crawly creatures. Cobwebs hung in the corners, showing gray and spidery in the wavering light of the lantern. My misgivings were heightened by the unpleasant smelly depths beneath me. A patient's sickening remark came into my mind. "Never let a snake crawl up into you," she said, looking fearfully behind her into the toilet bowl. "If you do, you'll never get it out." Only dire necessity made me use that pestilent outside toilet.

Hardy was chatting cheerfully. "We get spoiled at the hospital for this kind of thing. I'm so lucky to have steady work and steady pay! I help my folks out with money most months." The lantern threw spooky shadows in the darkness as we went back to the house.

Hardy threw the water in the basin out the door, and put fresh water from bucket and kettle out for me. She used it herself when I had washed my hands and face, and left it for morning. When water is carried in from an outdoor pump, it is conserved for communal use.

Hardy's parents and her brother were already in bed, having undressed while we were outside. Two backs were considerately turned in the bed next to us, but I was doubtful about the young boy. The gas lamp had been turned out so I couldn't see him behind the table. Maybe he hadn't reached the age of curiosity, but for once I wished I had a voluminous nightgown like my mother's. I had often seen her putting on or taking off clothes under it - at least I saw the motions she went through in protecting her modesty. Somehow I got out of my clothes and into my pajamas, and Hardy blew out the lantern. The smell of kerosene lingered in the air.

The strangeness of hearing the snuffling and snoring of the others kept me awake for awhile in the musty room, but all at once it was morning. Mr. Hardy was sitting on the far side of their bed and I realized I had to turn my back while he got dressed. When we heard Wilbert and his father go out the door, Hardy and I hurriedly got up and dressed before they came back in for the breakfast Mrs. Hardy was preparing.

No! Never would I want to live in these primitive conditions. The romance of the Cariboo country did not appeal to me. Not in the least.

CHAPTER ELEVEN

The day was fast approaching that would mark a full year since I had started working in the mental hospital. Examinations also fell in April and graduation exercises for the third-year students were set for the last week of the month. Marshall would be graduating, and Richmond. All of the student nurses except those on duty on the wards were expected to attend, in uniform.

"It's quite lah-de-dah," Marshall told us. "The big-wigs are in tuxedos and their wives wear evening dresses. There's an orchestra and a dance afterwards for the graduates and their guests. We get to invite one person besides our parents."

"Where do they hold it?" I asked. "There's no hall around here." I thought of the smelly gym in the Boys' Industrial School.

Marshall's answer was a surprise. "In ward H2's dayroom," she answered. "They clear out the furniture and the rugs in the center of the room and put in chairs for the student body and a platform. Guests sit around the edge. It's done up brown - flowers along the front of the platform, potted plants set around. And the graduates carry roses. I have already been given a long-sleeved blue uniform dress and two stripes to sew on my cap." She had worn one stripe for her senior year.

All the white pieces would have extra starch in them that week, even the students' bibs and aprons. I was looking forward to the graduation exercises.

After nearly 12 months on the wards I was feeling very self-confident. I had been on the tough ward, H4, for more than three months and thought I knew what to expect from the patients. In fact I had much to learn.

The first sign of trouble was a sharp jab in my ribs as I was unlocking the dayroom door to take the dormitory workers out to get their supplies from the utility room. I looked around quickly but the women's faces gave me no clue to the hostile action, and I decided it had been accidental.

The next morning the jab was repeated, again as my back was turned while I unlocked the door. I swung around sharply and scrutinized every face as the women filed past. They were all familiar workers except Miss Peck, who had just joined us.

I had been pleased when Miss Peck volunteered to work in the dormitory. Maudie, a regular worker and a good friend to the nurses, had been kept in bed with 'a touch of pneumonia' for the past week, and we kept her in her own bed instead of sending her to the Infirmary as she was such a good patient and followed the doctor's orders faithfully. I had asked for a volunteer to take her place and to everyone's surprise, Miss Peck came forward.

For the month she had been on H4, this sour-faced woman had been withdrawn and unfriendly. She seemed to exist in a state of watchful suspicion, refusing to speak and barely co-operating with the ward routine. Yet she was cosseted and given special privileges by Miss Steele. Word went around that Miss Peck had been a registered nurse in charge of a ward in a general hospital. Though her manner had not changed, her step forward to help in the dormitory while Maudie was sick was taken as a sign of improvement.

Miss Peck's bed was in the same room as Maudie's and she started by making it up, then pulled the others together in a desultory fashion before wandering out to another room. I had straightened Maudie's bed and made her comfortable, then went on to smooth out the spreads and fix hospital corners which Miss Peck had been at no pains to make correctly.

"That one isn't much help," Maudie said disdainfully when Miss Peck had gone. "What's she doing in here anyway? Stuck-up thing!"

"Maybe she's trying to get better," I said. "Doing something useful rather than sitting in the dayroom glaring at everybody." Maudie sniffed, unconvinced. I changed the subject.

"You look better, Maudie. Has Dr. Ryan said when you can sit up in the dayroom?"

"In a couple of days, he said, when my temperature stays normal. I think I just had a bad cold." Maudie's appetite was returning but she looked pale and not as rotund as usual. She was one of my most reliable workers and I would be glad to see her up and around again.

The next day there were two women in their beds, Maudie and Miss Peck who had complained to Miss Steele about a stomach ache. She didn't look sick. Perhaps it was a ruse to get out of dormitory work, though all she had to do was say she didn't want to do it. We didn't miss her lackadaisical help.

Again I was in their room, lining up beds, making sure they would meet with Miss Hicks' approval when she came in with Dr. Ryan. I was bent over re-doing a square corner when I sensed a rush behind me, and heard Maudie screaming, "Miss Lehman! Look out!" At that moment my uniform was ripped from neck to waist at the back.

I whirled around to fend off an infuriated Miss Peck, eyes blazing with hatred, face distorted and mouth twisted. "You deceitful bitch!" she spat at me. "You're the one who put me in here! I knew you had it in for me from the first! I'll see that you get yours, don't worry. You're the crazy one and I'm the nurse!"

She raved and cursed, tearing at my face and clothes. With both arms up to protect my face, as she was going for my eyes, I couldn't get hold of the mad woman. Maudie saved me.

Still weak from her illness, for she had been in bed for a week, Maudie had come to my aid. She leaped out of her bed and tried to get hold of Miss Peck's arms, but was thrown off easily. Maudie was still a heavyweight but the enraged woman was not to be prevented from her maniacal desire to punish me. It was a nightmare to be faced with such frenzied rage. Maudie kept at her from behind and the other workers and the ward staff came to my rescue, followed closely by a half dozen nurses from other wards. They soon subdued the crazed woman and led her away to Ward J.

"How did you know?" I half sobbed. "Was I screaming?"

"The dormitory workers came to tell us," Robertson said. "Come in the office and I'll see if I can pin you together enough so you can go upstairs for a uniform. Are you hurt?"

I was shaken and ashamed, but not hurt. Miss Peck had vented her fury on my uniform, which hung in shreds to my waist. Even the heavy starched bib was torn down the middle. Robertson sat me in a chair, for my knees were giving way and I was trembling. She tucked and pinned as much as she could to the starched collar that was still around my neck, pins dangling from it.

Miss Steele appeared at my elbow with a glass of water, and asked me to tell them about it. I remembered the jabs in my ribs and knew now it had been Miss Peck, so I started there, and I told them she had said I was responsible for her being in the hospital. "She hates me for some reason," I said, heart-broken. "I don't know why." I expected Miss Steele would be blaming me.

"There is no reason," Miss Steele exclaimed, a smile on her face. "She's transferred her delusions onto you, that's all. We're dealing with mental patients here, remember? You mustn't feel responsible for their irrationalities. Miss Peck has paranoidal tendencies and it could have been me she picked on - they often choose the one who's done the most for them. But you should have reported those jabs in the ribs. We'd have been watching for something unusual like her offering to work in the dormitories. I did think that was odd." I felt better to know that Miss Steele understood.

"Now I think you should go over to your room and lie down," the Supervisor said. "But you can't go like that! You'll have to go up to the OT and get another uniform. I'll phone Mrs. Rupert."

Robertson was tucking and pinning, and patting my shoulder. "Take the rest of the day off, Lehman," she said. "You had quite an ordeal. I'll make you a cup of tea first."

"Thanks, but I'd rather stay on the ward," I pleaded. "Please." I knew I'd break down and cry at the Home and felt I could keep control if I stayed on the ward. Besides, if I gave in now I might not be able to make myself come back. I needed company to bring my world back to normal. A lump in my throat thickened my voice, I said, "I don't want to be alone."

Robertson looked at me speculatively. "Well, go upstairs and get a uniform and we'll see. I'll send Hardy with you."

Hardy was just what I needed. She chatted companionably as we went up the stairs. "Golly, that Peck was planning this for some time, it looks like. Pretending she was sick and had to be in bed. I guess Maudie saved you, huh? If she'd been able to jump on Peck's back like she did on Big Campbell she'd have flattened her. I guess she's weak after the pneumonia. She wasn't terribly bad with it though, was she? Say, would you ever have believed sour old Peck could fight the way she did? And curse! I'll bet she was hated by her staff."

Hardy's chatter soothed and calmed me, and by the time we reached the sewing department I was able to endure Mrs. Rupert's fussy attention without breaking down.

"Dear, dear! Your uniform is in rags. Except for the apron and belt, and the collar. We can take the cuffs off too, they're all right. Now you leave it to me. Just come into my office and take that one off. I've put one out for you that should be the right size. We're so busy this time of year, with new probationers again. I looked in your laundry compartment and there was a bib there. So that's yours. Let's see - that uniform fits just right. Suppose you put a name tag in it and keep it. I'll make another - it was either one for you now or later, so it may as well be now. Dear, dear! Another uniform to cut out!" We left her in her usual dither expressing her usual complaints.

I was still strung up when we returned to the ward but slipped into the dayroom where Robertson found me. Hardy had told me that Carmack had taken over the dormitory. "If you're determined to stay, Lehman, just take it easy." Robertson patted my arm again and went back to the office.

Dr. Ryan arrived shortly, attended by the three high-placed nurses, and made an unprecedented stop in front of me.

"I hear you had quite an experience this morning," he said, his piercing gaze upon me. "We'll keep Miss Peck on ward J until she's quite recovered. But you don't have to stay on the ward now. You can have the rest of the day off, you know." Miss Steele was nodding her head. She had briefed him well.

The lump in my throat prevented me from speaking, but I shook my head, wishing I could fall through the floor with those four pairs of eyes on me. Dr. Ryan said no more, but I thought I saw respect in his eyes and that told me I was doing the right thing. He moved on, and the other three followed with smiles on their faces. An encouraging look from Miss Hicks raised my spirits.

Queenie was berating Dr. Ryan as usual at the end of the room. It struck me that I was not the only one who was the object of paranoidal hatred. My self-respect began to return, and with it my inner composure. My world was returning to normal, but I had learned a lesson I had needed amongst these unreliable women.

Human behavior was unpredictable in the normal world too. When Fraser had left to be married, she had invited Gladwin and me to visit her. Glad was the first to look her up, and she came back with incredible news. Her face was a study in astonishment and she burst out as soon as she came into our room, "Guess what! Fraser's husband is in a wheelchair! A paraplegic!" She stuttered over the unfamiliar word.

"He works four hours a day - I don't know what or where. He's picked up in a van. So Fraser and I had a chance to talk and she told me George had polio when he was quite young. Imagine! Marrying a man in a wheelchair! And she never said a word!"

"Why on earth would she tie herself to a man in a wheelchair?" I wondered. "Do you think she's any happier?"

"Well, you know Fraser. It seemed to me she complains as much as ever, but she waits on George hand and foot. And you know, he's good-looking all right, but he's not that nice to her. I wouldn't want to be ordered around like that."

Glad and I went together the next time and I met Fraser's husband. George had a strong handshake but I was uneasy in his company, for Gladwin was right, he did expect Fraser to fetch and carry for him. After he went off to work Fraser made tea for us and we sat down to talk. Fraser launched into a round of complaints about life with a disabled man.

"You've no idea how much time I spend wheeling him around," she said. "When we go to the corner store to shop, he has to hold the groceries and I push the chair. And before next summer," she paused and lowered her eyelids, "There'll be one more to look after."

"You mean," Gladwin glanced at me, "You're having a baby?"

As the years went on Fraser had three babies. We saw her wheeling her husband around while she was pregnant. Then she pushed the wheelchair with George holding the baby in his lap. Next she was pregnant again, pushing the wheelchair with the two of them in it. Then the first little toddler was hanging on to the wheelchair while George held a baby again. We couldn't believe it when she became pregnant again.

"Is she crazy?" I asked. "Or does she like having people feel sorry for her?"

"That's it, Lehman!" Oliver said. We were in the staff dining room. "That's exactly it. Fraser is the martyr type." But Fraser was kind, I thought. I remembered her gentle treatment of the women on F4, and Fraser was a good wife and mother. Though not the happiest person to live with.

Meanwhile we had attended our first graduation exercises as part of the student body that marched in, class by class, to the chairs in the middle of the room. Our first-year class sat at the very back, then the second years in the middle, then the graduating class in front of them. In the very front rows were the post-graduate students, general hospital graduates who were finishing a course in psychiatric nursing. They had been on the wards as onlookers, more or less, and they didn't have the long hours that we had. Now they would receive a certificate and be on the lookout for a job again.

The march-in must have been impressive, everyone in clean starched uniforms, the graduates carrying large bouquets of roses. The orchestra provided appropriate music, the guests and the platform party standing until all were in place. Then the strains of 'O Canada' to which everyone added their voices as they sang along marked the beginning of the program. Now we could settle back and enjoy the proceedings.

The Chairman was Mr. P. Walker, Deputy Minister of Health in the provincial government. The hospital Chaplain gave the Invocation. Then Dr. Sedgewick, a well-known professor of English at the University of British Columbia, addressed the graduating class. He was witty and scholarly, making the uncertain future of young people in the depressed 30s appear to depend on their inner resources in troubled times. At least the mental hospital graduates had continued employment ahead, if they wished to stay on, and most of them did.

The printed program showed that the diplomas were being given out by Dr. A.L. Crease, Superintendent of the Mental Hospital. I had never set eyes on the great man until this evening. His office was in the Acute Building and he lived in the largest of the doctors' houses up on the hill. A man who held the highest position in this large complex, his importance was reflected in his ponderous appearance. Miss Hicks was dwarfed at his side, but her dignity matched his as she pinned a bar with a pendant medal to the bib of each graduate, and congratulated them. Her pride in her nurses and in the program she had formulated along the lines of general hospital nursing education showed in every smile she gave.

Of the 14 graduates, two were leaving to be married. It was not possible to hold a job after marriage, and nobody expected it. Two salaries in one household when so many homes had none? Never!

The post-graduate nurses went up for their certificates, then a rustle around the room preceded the most important part of the ceremony. Who would receive the special award, the Deputy Minister's medal?

Mrs. Walker, elegant in a long dress, rose to make the presentation. The Chairman paused, intensifying the suspense. Even the recipient had not been told.

"The Deputy Minister's wife will present the award for general proficiency to...Hazel Marshall!" My friend was judged the most efficient nurse in her class! Of course she would be! Loud clapping broke out. It was a popular choice.

I clapped harder than the rest as Marshall went up to receive her prize, her head thrust forward from the rest of her body as usual, as if she couldn't wait to get there. She stood straight and flushed with pride as the prestigious medal was pinned on her bib.

Prizes for highest marks in each class were next. Richmond had achieved that honor in third year, as Marshall had told me she would, having been consistently top of the class right through. Oliver was given the award she had earned for the highest marks in first year.

The orchestra played 'God Save the King', then the student body marched out leaving the graduates to receive congratulations from friends and relatives. We could have returned for the dance to follow if we had partners waiting for us in the rotunda, but Glad and I did not and we went back to the Nurses' Home.

"Only two more years for us!" Gladwin said, taking her uniform off and carefully laying it over a chair for the next day.

"Do you think we'll be here that long?" For some reason the impressive ceremonies had saddened me. They were a copy of the general hospital graduation exercises, but a psychiatric nurse's meticulous training and arduous studies meant nothing away from Essondale. The 14 graduates tonight had little choice but to stay on the wards 'until things opened up.' There was always the hope that the economic situation would improve soon. After all, 'things' had been tough in employment for four years already. Little did we know!

While we had been waiting to march in, I had overheard one of the graduating class say that she had applied at the Vancouver General Hospital for nurses' training and was told that no credit was given for her three years training at Essondale. She would have to start as a lowly probationer. "But I'm going to do it," she said firmly. "The lectures should be easy after all we've had here." Reports came back to us that our graduate did indeed excel in bedside nursing and in tests, and graduated with the highest marks in her class. She eventually became Charge of one of the wards in the general hospital.

Unless a psychiatric nurse was assigned to the male or female infirmary during her training, and not every one was, her experience in bedside nursing was practically nil. Our knowledge of the mentally ill was extensive but there were no psychiatric wards in general hospitals at that time so our prospects of using that learning anywhere but at Essondale were non-existent.

Miss Hicks' high standards for her nursing staff were recognized by Dr. Ryan and his associates. The Medical Superintendent expressed his confidence in a report that read, 'The trained medical and nursing staff, collaborating with the technicians of the laboratory, dispensary, and X-Ray department is capable of giving patients the same treatment rendered in a general hospital.' It was years before general hospitals acknowledged our training by allowing for it when a psychiatric graduate sought admission to general hospital training.

CHAPTER TWELVE

Now we were second year students, with a whole summer free of lectures ahead of us. For the first time my roommate and I were on different shifts. Gladwin stayed on days, and I spent my second summer at Essondale on night duty. Walford, still a lone individual, and I were on F2, one of the 'good' wards.

Because I had been taken on a week ahead of Walford, it fell to me to make the count night and morning, and to write up the ward reports. Walford was still wrapped up in her own little cocoon. She would answer, though briefly, when spoken to. The prospect of having to initiate all conversation for the next four months was rather daunting. "I'll be haunting your room," I told Oliver and Hammond, who were also on nights. "Marshall is still on days, too."

Walford had turned out to be a very efficient nurse, so we had no problems on F2 that we couldn't handle. The senile women had to be assisted somewhat, though they had been spaced throughout the different rooms and there were usually kind souls nearby to help them along. Walford and I looked up clean clothes and supervised the stripping of beds on laundry days, made sure the shower schedule was followed, and settled arguments over personal belongings. The patients looked after themselves pretty well on this ward.

Like Queenie with her capacious black bag stuffed with treasures, many of the women carried some sort of handbag with their comb, hairbrush, toothbrush and whatever cosmetics they still owned, in it. When we had to empty a bag out onto a bed to settle a dispute, we found strange things which the woman held onto in spite of their utter uselessness. Empty perfume bottles and cold cream jars, a comb without teeth, old laundry lists, broken jewelry. Some carried letters, which they never looked at. But you couldn't take a thing away from them. These were their links to the past.

"Check Freda's bag when something is missing," day staff told us. "She's a kleptomaniac. She'll swipe things off your table, too." Freda muttered dire threats but allowed us to take the stolen article back to the owner. There would always be something else to slip into her bag, whether she could use it or not. Taking things was a compulsion with Freda.

The hours to midnight went quickly enough, with the doctor's visit and Walford relieving the top floor staff for the one meal we had while on duty, and I went for my own dinner when she came back. The early morning hours were the worst for staying awake.

Walford and I were both great readers but had to have something else to do. We both knitted, and eventually I brought some crocheting, working on some lace for my hope chest. Walford watched me awhile and then shyly asked, "Would you show me how to crochet?"

This opened a new dimension in our relationship, for Walford, once having made the first move, was then able to ask me for help with her new activity when she needed it. It was a start, at least, and probably led to the release of long pent-up emotions which had been stifling her.

One night after being off and not getting a day's sleep, I stopped work and said in a low voice, "I have to talk or I'll be dropping off. What do you do on your days off, Walford?"

Walford's expression altered. Her face twisted as if pained, and she blinked a couple of times, holding back tears. "All the work that's been waiting for me since the last time I was home. You wouldn't expect my brothers to lay a hand to anything, would you?" She bent her head and blew her nose, then straightened up and began to talk. She was so full of hurts that it all tumbled out in a jumble, from the favoritism shown her two brothers by their mother to the unwanted attentions she received from her father.

A picture emerged of a family centered on the males. Walford, the only girl, had an older brother, Jack, and a younger brother, Jerry. Her mother waited on them hand and foot and made their sister do the same. Because she was a girl, she was expected to help in the house but also do the chores that could have fallen to the boys, even mowing the lawn.

"Jack and Jerry could go out to play ball or ride their bicycles, while I washed dishes and cleaned up after them. Every Saturday I had to scrub the kitchen floor, and change the beds - theirs too, of course, and tidy up after them. They scattered stuff around on purpose, I know they did." The boys and their father were served first at the table and if they took all of anything she and her mother did without. "Maybe she didn't mind, with her ideas about men first, but I did!"

And Jack was mean, downright mean. He tormented his sister with a form of low-minded teasing that she was helpless against, having found at an early age that her mother would not come to her rescue. "Even when he punched me in the stomach so I was gasping for breath, and she was right there, he got away with it," Walford's eyes were sparking fire now. "I don't know which was worse, being punched in the stomach or on my breasts, after I was old enough to have them. You can get cancer from blows on the breasts, can't you, Lehman?" I had heard you could, but I shook my head, and said I hoped not.

"I knew I couldn't punch him back, the big bully. He's always been twice my size. Oh, he's mean! The teasing, like saying I was fat and stupid and ugly - anything to make me feel awful. And Mother never told him to stop. Her darling son could do no wrong."

"What about your dad?" I asked, sick at the thought of all Walford had disclosed. Yet she had lots more to tell.

"Oh, he wasn't around, most of the time. Jack knew when he could get mean all right. But, Dad..." She stopped, wiped the tears from her eyes, and her face hardened. "Dad had his own kind of tormenting. I guess he thought it was all right to treat a little girl like a toy but it made me darned uncomfortable. Oh, I loved it to begin with, Daddy's game. But I cringe now when I think of how he showed me off. I guess it started about as soon as I could walk. Anyway when I was in my nightie, ready for bed, he'd tickle my bare tummy. Especially when there was company. I'd run up to him lifting my nightie, he'd tickle and laugh, and I'd run away. When I got old enough I noticed a look of disgust on a woman's face - her husband was laughing of course, and I became ashamed to think I'd been made to show myself off."

"Was your mother there?" I asked, but I knew the answer. She was. Walford now showed more signs of distress, but she was determined to get it all out. When her breasts began to grow her father would come up behind her and feel them, with both hands, one on each breast. "I'd have to pull away from him, and no matter how I'd beg him or yell at him to stop, he'd do it again. And don't ask me, my mother knew all about that too. It's just as if they both thought I was a plaything for my father. I hated it! He did that for years."

At that time, in her early adolescence, Jack started a new form of sadistic teasing. For some reason she couldn't fathom, as she knew how mean he was, Jack was popular with the girls, and he had a following of boys who thought he was smart, too. So there were a number of kids around in the school playground when he threw his verbal blow.

That morning when Walford was getting dressed, with her door closed over but not shut tight, Jack gave it a kick as he went by and said, "Haw haw" or something like that at seeing her not dressed. She was sitting on the bed putting on her stockings so she figured he couldn't have seen very much, and forgot about it. But at recess he found her on the schoolground and said, "Why don't you tell everybody what you were doing to yourself in your room this morning?"

Every eye was on her, and she heard some snickers. "I was just getting dressed," she said hotly, but she was beaten. His insinuation was too clear, and the kids drifted off, leaving her red-faced - and innocent. "That was a typical Jack remark," Walford said indignantly. "I didn't have a friend, ever. Jack was there ahead of me."

"What about Jerry?" I asked. "Couldn't he see how things were?"

"Oh yes, he saw how the boys were favored and he liked it that way. He wasn't as mean as Jack, but he followed his example the way I was treated like a servant for them. Mother even saw to it that I cleaned their shoes, along with dad's. Just to show you what it's like at our house, since I've been working here I have to hand over half of my pay every month. 'For room and board' even though I'm here most of the time and do housework when I'm home. But did the boys ever hand over a cent? Nosiree, not them! Jack helps at the boatyard where Dad works and has since he was 14, but he gets to keep his pay. And now he's married - but wait, I have to tell you what he tried with me one time." I had a feeling I'd rather not hear it, but she went on. Telling must have been a liberation for her, a release of pain that was borne alone too long.

Walford had been in the woodshed, picking up an armload to take inside. She was about 14. "Jack came up behind me and pushed me to the floor, he was on top of me with his hand up my skirt, on my legs. I was menstruating and I gasped, 'You can't! I'm wearing a rag!' and by that time he'd felt it. He got up looking disgusted and he didn't try that again. I bet he did with other girls, for now he's brought a 16-year old girl home and they've been married. She was pregnant, of course. And what do you think mother does?" She paused, as if she couldn't believe it herself. "She takes her daughter-in-law breakfast in bed!"

After her one outburst Walford said nothing further about her home life, except to say a little later that Jack and his bride had found a house to rent, and Jack had been taken on steady at the boatyard now that he was a married man. Walford started going out with one of the attendants the next year and they were married a couple of years later. I was glad she found someone who put her first, as this man obviously did. Then because she lived in Coquitlam and I lived in New Westminster, we lost track of each other.

Our second year psychology course emphasized the point that no one should try to bear his troubles alone. "I'm not saying you're supposed to tell the world," Dr. Gee said. "But if there is just one person you can talk to, your mental health will be better than if you bottle things up inside."

Before summer was over Richmond had given her notice. She would be teaching in Vavenby, a sawmill town on the Canadian National Railway line north of Kamloops. "I applied to 40 schools, from ads in the paper," she said. "I got one answer. So that's it. I'll get experience, anyway, and I might get back to the city some day."

Richmond's letters were full of descriptions of a different kind of life in the remote region near the Rockies. "There's a two-roomed school," she wrote. "I have the upper grades, 5 to 8, which means there are some big boys and girls in my room. There's electricity but we get water from a pump in the yard. Two outdoor toilets, pretty rough for a city girl! The primary teacher and I have a teacherage by the schoolgrounds, which I like. The winters will get colder here than they ever get on the Coast."

She described the rodeo held at the end of summer, practically the first entertainment she attended. Dances were held in the community hall every Friday night. On Wednesday and Saturday nights there were movies. "Sound hasn't arrived here yet," she wrote. "The postmaster's wife plays the organ, and creates the sound effects - thunder, rifle shots, horses' hoofs - for the pictures. Wednesday night is amateur night and I'm learning quite a lot about the people here, seeing the acts they put on. Saturday they run a serial, the 'Perils of Pauline' where Pauline is always left gagged and tied, lying on the railway track with a train coming, or hanging by one hand to a branch over a cliff, to get you back the next week."

She described the school events. "We're practising already for the Christmas concert. We've had deep snowfalls and everybody skis. A schoolbus - some of the kids are brought in from 20 miles away - picks up the older ones on Friday noon every week and takes them up to the ski runs. I'm learning, too! And they've cleared a skating rink by the pump in the schoolyard, and pump water into it last thing after school, and have a fresh surface of ice by morning. The kids skate before school, at recess, and after school. There's a pile of skates in the coatroom, and the kids just put on whatever fits. You should see the rosy cheeks up here! The girls have beautiful complexions. There's a lot of horseback riding, too."

Richmond wrote she was being invited into the homes, and her description of one visit was hilarious. Mr. and Mrs. Berry had no children in school, or grandchildren, as their son and daughter had moved elsewhere when they married. They were in their 80s, having just celebrated 60 years of marriage. "Though they haven't been together 60 years," the postmaster's wife told Richmond. "She moved in with a guide for a couple of years. She's a great hunter." Mrs. Berry eventually returned to her husband and all seemed to be well.

In fact, Mr. Berry turned out to be an inordinately fond husband, proud of everything his wife had done. "The guide episode excluded, I would suppose," Richmond wrote. "It certainly wasn't mentioned." First he showed their visitor the garden. "She dug it all," Mr. Berry said, jabbing a thumb in his wife's direction. "Planted the vegetables, all kinds, and hoed and weeded." "Pickled and canned, too," Mrs. Berry added, nodding her head.

"There's lots put into the cellar," the husband went on. "I'll show you." He lifted a trap door on the floor of the large porch, and Richmond saw a deep pit of considerable size, with a ladder going down into it. There were piles of turnips, potatoes, squash, and probably more in a space about eight feet square.

His face beaming, the old gentleman said, "She dug this, too. Every bit of it, while I was working in the woods." Mrs. Berry, about five feet tall and slightly built, nodded. It did seem incredible.

Then Mr. Berry pointed to a set of antlers mounted on the wall of the porch. "The biggest spread of any that've been shot in the Kamloops district," he said proudly. "She got it." Every time he said 'she' he underlined it with his voice, and nodded to his wife.

They lived in an eight-foot wide trailer, one of the first of the trailer homes. It was maybe 20 feet long, and the living room took most of that space. Richmond, who is tall, had to dodge antlers mounted on both sides - deer, elk, antelope. "She killed all of 'em." Of course, a black bear rug was on the floor. "Yep, she got that, too."

Mrs. Berry seated herself behind a projector all set up for showing pictures of a horseback trip she had been on, last summer. "With a party, you know, and a guide." Why, she would be 80! Or awfully close. What a remarkable woman she was.

The scenery must have been beautiful, for the ride started at Mt. Robson and went into the Rockies, but the picture bounced so much that Richmond thought there must be something wrong with the machine. Mrs. Berry's next remark explained the rocking motion. "These were taken from horseback," she said. "Beautiful country! And we had a wonderful guide!" Richmond thought she saw Mrs. Berry slant an enigmatic glance at her husband, whose air of pride didn't waver. A remarkable couple.

Richmond taught for three years at Vavenby, and told us she

had received four proposals of marriage. "Many of the wives there had been schoolteachers," she said. "There was a continual turnover of teachers, because of course they couldn't stay on when they got married." The Second World War changed that, very quickly. Soon the School Boards would be asking married teachers to return to the classrooms, and they made better teachers for having raised children of their own.

Richmond moved to a school in the Fraser Valley, closer to her family. She became principal of a large elementary school, a very good one. She never married. "I've had hundreds of children pass through my hands," she said. "It's a very rewarding life."

My second summer at Essondale was a very hot one, and we spent as much time as possible in the pool at the Red Bridge. Ferrier was on nights, too, and I saw her there, creating a sensation in a bathing suit composed of a brief bra and shorts. One-piece suits were the only kind we had previously seen. The boys were ecstatic, the girls jealous. We couldn't have matched Ferrier in bra size, anyway, even if we'd had two-piece suits.

Ferrier paid little attention to me, and I was taken by surprise one morning when she came to my room. "Say, Lehman, how about helping me bring our bikes back from the Wild Duck Inn?" She and Dunbar had bicycled out to the beer parlor on the Pitt River and their bikes were still there. "We got a ride back. We can start out sharp at three, and we'll be back in time for second supper. Will you do it?" Her foxy face could be very pleasant when she wanted a favor. "We can cycle back."

I protested, "I can't ride a bicycle. I've never tried." The Wild Duck Inn was about four miles out, quite a hike on a hot day.

"Oh, it's easy. I'll help you get started. See you at three."

We arrived at the Inn a little after four. Ferrier got the two bicycles and looked at my wide pajama legs. I was wearing beach pajamas with a halter top and the widest flared bottoms imaginable. Ferrier advised me to tuck them up above the knees. Then I tried to hop on while she ran alongside holding the bike.

It was impossible. I couldn't keep my balance. We were on a grassy verge with enough traffic on the graveled road so that we had to stay off it. I'd get going, then a car coming toward me unnerved me and I toppled. My rolled up pajama bottoms kept falling down and I had to stop in case the material caught in the gears. We were both sweating and the hot sun blazed down.

"I just can't stay up, Ferrier," I said. "I'll walk the bike back. You don't have to wait for me." Ferrier, of course, rode easily.

To Ferrier's credit she stayed with me and walked her bicycle too. She was wearing a short-sleeved cotton blouse and summer slacks. I had nothing to protect my arms and back.

It was almost six o'clock when we wheeled the bicycles up to the Home. "Just time for a shower and get into our uniforms. Put some salve on your arms and back, Lehman. They look pretty red."

The shower stung, and I knew I was burned. All I had to put on my shoulders, which were the worst, was vaseline. When I put on my uniform the starched collar hurt unbearably. I looked around for something to pad it with.

As if on cue, Ferrier appeared with a handful of sanitary pads. "Here, let me put these under your collar, Lehman. You're going to have an uncomfortable night. Say, where did you get that pretty ring?" My opal ring was on my dresser, as I didn't wear it at work. It had belonged to my grandmother, and was my prized possession. Ferrier picked it up and admired the changing colors of blue and purple, and I'm quite sure she left it there. Almost quite sure. The ring was missing a few days later. Perhaps that was my thanks for helping Ferrier get the bicycles home. That, and a sunburn.

Ferrier returned to her former manner with me, which suited both of us. An incident in which she was involved occurred on Sullivan's ward some time later. Ferrier wasn't on staff but was relieving that day and she came into the dispensary when Sullivan was getting something out for me. Sullivan stopped to speak to her friend. I knew they had been chummy lately.

"How was your date last night, Ferrier?" she asked. Her green eyes rested on the foxy features facing her and the same expression came into both faces, a knowing, secret look.

"Just so-so," said Ferrier nonchalantly. She held one hand at her waist, palm up. "Lots of action from here up." Then she turned her hand over so it was palm down. "But nothing from here down."

Their shared laugh excluded me. How fortunate that my sore feet had kept me from going out with Sullivan that time! Keith would have seen that I hadn't, anyway. It seemed so long ago

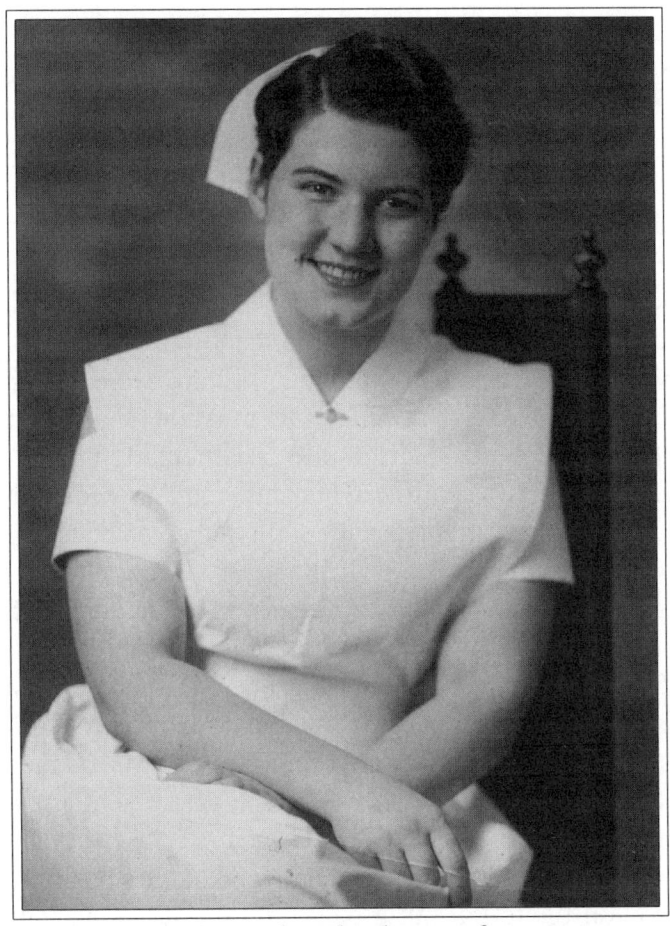

The author in her third year of nursing.

CHAPTER THIRTEEN

My ward assignments in my second year were even more challenging than those I had already been given. After I came off nights I spent six months on the Women's Admitting Ward, in the Acute Building. The only wards with nurses on them in the center building were E4, Admitting, on the top floor, and E2, the Men's Infirmary, on the main floor. Of the ten nurses who walked the longer distance, past the Female Chronic Building, six of us took the elevator to the top floor.

The rest of the wards in the Acute Building were men's wards, staffed by attendants. We never saw them while on duty, either the male patients or the attendants, unless a particularly violent admission called for more strength than our staff could provide. Then two stalwart men appeared and often the sight of them subdued a recalcitrant woman very quickly.

In spite of the small number of nurses in the Acute Building, we had a dining room to ourselves. I missed the sociability of meeting friends from other wards, and the atmosphere was more formal as we were joined by the ward supervisors, Miss Seymour on Admitting and Miss Ashcroft from the Men's Infirmary, as well as the Charge Nurses from these wards. A male patient, as efficient and quiet as Mrs. May, served us.

The supervisors were pleasant enough but their positions of authority couldn't help but put a constraint on our conversation. In their immaculate white uniforms they represented the Administrative staff. And to sit down with Milner, my Charge Nurse who gave me my orders, very effectively curbed my usually loquacious tongue.

Otherwise E4 was a welcome diversion. Patients coming in might overcome their problems and we worked in an air of expectation that gave vibrancy to the days. The hopelessness of the Female Chronic Building had weighed on my spirits more than I realized until I came to E4. Before the days of insulin and electric shock treatments, and the advent of mood-altering drugs other than sedatives, the only therapy was physiotherapy, in its many forms. Very few women improved enough, once they were transferred to the Women's Building, to be discharged; cynical older nurses stated flatly that most of those who did go home would be back sooner or later. Working in the Acute Building, though apart from my friends, was an agreeable change.

Patients who came to E4 were more likely to improve, and go home. There was Sheila, who was a secretary with a good job. She was admitted in a highly excited state, fighting off imagined medieval soldiers who, she felt, were subjecting her to the tortures of the rack, fingernail piercing, boiling oil and other evil practices. Hydrotherapy, sedatives and time worked their magic, and Sheila became the pet of the ward. She made tea for the nurses and we poured her a cup to have with us, and found her to be a charming, polite woman. She was discharged before the four-month period, considered the point-of-no-return if improvement had not been made, was up.

Some of the admissions were in a very depressed condition, and I had personal insight into one of these shortly after I came on the ward. Milner, the Charge Nurse, called me into the office when I had been there a week. "Lehman, you're to go into New Westminster with the police officers to pick up a new patient. Get your cape and wait at the entrance downstairs. They should be along any minute."

This was a new experience. The police car drew up, I was invited into the front seat and the three of us chatted companionably on the 20-minute drive into town.

The driver stopped on a quiet street in a residential area. Both men went into the house, leaving me in the car. They came out almost immediately holding a sobbing young girl by the arm, and put her into the car. I was now officially in charge of the patient and sat with her in the back seat, distressed by her insistent weeping. She would not be comforted, shrinking into her corner and dabbing at her eyes with a sodden handkerchief.

In a few minutes we drew up at a medical building where we went into a doctor's waiting room, where the girl and I sat down. The four of us were the only people there, but it was five minutes before the office door opened and a short, stout, bespectacled man appeared. He looked around, and asked, "Which one is the patient?"

With a resigned look one of the policemen indicated the only person not in uniform, the red-eyed girl with her face averted, unable to control her tears. The doctor motioned the girl into his office. She didn't seem to understand, and he took her by her arm and led her in, closing the door behind them.

Shortly the door opened and he handed the policeman a signed permission to admit the girl to the mental hospital. The family doctor must have signed earlier, as two signatures were required.

We made the return journey in silence punctuated by the sobs of the young girl, who could not have been older than I was. Her hair had become wet around her face and hung untidily in strands that she kept pushing back from her puffed eyes and damp cheeks.

"What on earth is the matter with her?" I asked Milner, after the girl had been given the required bath, sedated and put to bed. "Do you have her history yet?" On this ward we had some chance of learning something of the background of admissions, if the Charge told us. We were not allowed to read the records, otherwise.

"There's not much help here, to explain her depression. Poor family, father not working, on relief. Or maybe that is the explanation! The future doesn't have much to offer her."

Many people faced these conditions and survived without breaking down. That had been a point Dr. Gee had made, in lectures, that there seems to be a predisposition to mental illness in some cases.

We were also told that if conditions that led to a breakdown remained the same, a patient who recovers can go home from the hospital and become ill again. There were mental health workers who visited the homes to help the family of a mentally ill person, to try to prepare them to change whatever brought on the breakdown.

Perhaps this young girl would recover and be able to return home. But if she was subjected to the same environment that upset her in the first place, what hope was there?

On another occasion I was asked to accompany a woman on a

visit to her dentist in town. There was a dentist on staff at the hospital but Mrs. Stanley's family wanted her to go to her own dentist.

"Pick up money for bus fares at the office downstairs," Miss Ashcroft told me. "The bus will be coming by in 20 minutes, and the schedule allows you to get back for supper. Wear ordinary clothes - don't wear your uniform."

This was an unusual assignment too. I had some qualms about the trip but it proved to be uneventful. Mrs. Stanley was uncommunicative and did not respond to my attempts at conversation, but she gave me no trouble. "I know Mrs. Stanley well," the dentist said. "You don't have to come in with her." I read magazines in the waiting room for an hour, and remembered my last visit to a dentist uneasily. What should I, what could I have done?

Since we had moved into town I hadn't been to a dentist so I had picked one within walking distance of our house. Many dentists, and some doctors, didn't have any help in the office, doing their own billing and keeping records. That was not at all unusual in the 30s. So it was in this office.

The dentist talked steadily while working on my teeth, mostly about his new boat that slept four. I was unable to answer him and wasn't even listening closely, distracted by the drill. I thought I heard him say how pleasant it was on Burrard Inlet and up Indian Arm, and wouldn't I enjoy that kind of outing? With my mouth full of instruments, his fingers, and cotton wads around my teeth, I gargled agreement. Who wouldn't? To me it was a hypothetical question.

When the fillings were finished and the wads removed, the talkative dentist fitted a brush onto his drill and slathered it with cleaning paste. "I'll just clean these off now," he said, and proceeded to run the drill over my front teeth.

The drill slipped and paste spattered on the front of my blouse and on my skirt as well. I could wash the blouse but the skirt worried me. "Oh, don't worry. I'll wipe it off," the dentist said. He took a cloth and dabbed at the spots on my blouse.

He whipped one hand underneath my knee-length skirt, which in the days of stockings and garters meant his hand was in direct contact with my bare skin. He was wiping at my skirt with the cloth.

I thrust my clasped hands on my lap and held them down tightly, to prevent him going any further. He now lifted the skirt material as if all he was interested in was getting it clean. I had my doubts, and got out of the chair as soon as he withdrew his hand. Without saying a word - I didn't know what he had in mind but I felt queasy - I picked up my coat and walked out. When a bill arrived I ignored it, and he didn't send another. I never wanted to see him again.

The only person I told about it was my mother, and her quick stare and unfeeling comment kept me from confiding in anyone else. "You must have encouraged him," she said.

No wonder Hammond couldn't tell her mother about her father's unwanted attentions. Women didn't trust women, it seemed. Not even, or especially not, their own daughters.

One of the new probationers on E4 was Margaret Lord. She and her sister Ella had come into the probies' dormitory together in the spring, and when rooms were available they had moved down next door to us. On different wards, they were each known as 'Lord', but in the Home we had to use their first names, or bog down entirely. Ella told us how a girl who started after they did, hearing 'Ella' and 'Margaret', announced loudly, "My name is Beryl. That's Burr-yl, not Bare-yl. I don't want to hear any 'barrels' around here." She didn't. She was called by her last name, like everybody else - except Ella and Margaret.

Ella was the older, and when we knew her better we no longer noticed her habit of screwing up her face so that her eyes were almost closed when she spoke, slowly, as if considering every word. That was Ella, and she was a really nice girl.

Margaret was the good-looking one. Her rosy cheeks were a contrast to Ella's pasty complexion, and her dark hair was trained into deep waves while Ella let her mousy-brown hair hang straight. Margaret was always smiling. Ella was the serious one. They both had low, gentle voices, exactly like their mother's, I was to learn.

Margaret had been on E4 ever since her orientation week, and was moved to another ward two months after I arrived on E4. In that time we became great friends, and the first time we had the same day off she asked me to come home with her. They lived on a farm in Maple Ridge, on the far side of the Pitt River.

We took the bus out and walked the half-mile to their place. A flock of turkeys in the front yard gave me a scare, pressing in on me, their repulsive-looking red wattles quivering as they gobbled fiercely at me. "Just keep going, Lehman. They won't hurt you," Margaret smiled at my fright. I was not acquainted with turkey ways, as we had never raised them, but I held my suitcase out to ward them off and was relieved to reach the safety of the porch.

The front door opened right into the living room so I met Mr. Lord and the girls' three brothers first. Mr. Lord was reading the newspaper with his feet up on a stool, and he waved it at us while he was saying hello. "Those Dionne quintuplets are getting real cute. Look at this! Five of them and you couldn't tell one from the other!" There had been daily coverage of the progress of the baby girls born in the province of Ontario. We studied the latest picture, awed by the phenomenon of their survival against all the odds.

Mr. Lord put his pipe back between his teeth and resumed reading the paper, his bald head shining under the light. Margaret introduced me to her three brothers, and they acknowledged me with a nod. Two were older than the girls, so shy they seldom spoke in my presence. They mumbled something about having to go out on some farm chores and left us. The younger brother was doing his homework at the large round table in the dining area of the long room. He looked more like Margaret than the other two, who resembled their father even to the balding heads. He was just as bashful, though, merely nodding at us and keeping his eyes on his books.

We found Mrs. Lord in the kitchen, washing the dishes. "My hands are wet, my dears, so I didn't come out. I knew you'd be in here." She was a gentle woman, slow in her movements and never finished with her work. I loved her on sight, and she became a second mother to me.

Margaret took over the dishpan, urging her mother to go in and sit down, while I dried the dishes. Mrs. Lord stayed in the kitchen, tidying up and talking to us. She was genuinely interested in our work. "I didn't want the girls to apply there, but there's nothing for them here," she said, her face troubled. I blithely assured her the work was not dangerous and that we enjoyed it, and that companionship among the girls was great.

Upstairs in her room, Margaret told me, "Ella and I hated to leave mother with all the work here, but there's not much money coming in from the farm, and no work for the boys."

As I came to know this family better through the years, my heart ached for Mrs. Lord. Three sons at home made Mr. Lord's work much easier, but no thought was given by any of them to the work they made for their mother. Mrs. Lord continued to cook their meals, wash and iron their clothes, and clean up after the four men for all of her life, until she died at age 82, for the three shy sons never married.

Saddest of all was the information that came my way years later. Talking to a friend who also had lived in Maple Ridge, the Lords were mentioned. "It was a shame about those boys," she said. "They were sexually molested by a teacher. He was fired by the School Board but he moved up country and was soon teaching again. A shame."

Margaret and Ella married and left for homes of their own, unlike the boys. They were bald like their father by the time they were 30, which didn't help their shyness any. They had no prospects, except to work on their father's farm and so they remained bachelors.

The boys became accustomed to seeing me around, and joined our activities around their home. Margaret and Ella brought young people in and the boys played baseball with us in one of the farm fields. When one of the girls played the piano in the living room and we all gathered around to sing, they joined us and sang, too. But if a neighbor lad took us to the beach at White Rock, or to a picnic in Stanley Park, the brothers could not be persuaded to come along. Mr. and Mrs. Lord smiled indulgently and told us to run along without them. We likely wouldn't be back in time for them to do the chores, anyway.

I never saw one of them lift a hand to help their mother in the house. Not once.

Ella and Margaret came to the Saturday night dances with us that winter. There we were all called by our first names by the other dancers, though last names came naturally among ourselves. Stan wasn't at the dances this year. "He's at a relief camp on the Hope-Princeton trail," his friends said. "And he hates it. The foreman has them clearing trails that will never be used. He'll probably cut out in the spring."

"Relief camp!" exploded Tim. "Miles from anywhere! Nothing to do but work, eat and sleep. Big pay! Yeah, 20 lousy cents a day! Say, have you heard about Russia? They need tractor drivers, and mechanics. I'd sure like to go, but..." His voice faded. How would he get the fare?

Bob, who was 'between' jobs, spoke up. "Chester, you had work in Calgary last summer, didn't you? How come you didn't stay there? Weren't you delivering coal?"

Chester laughed bitterly. "Now there's a dirty job! Filling sacks at the coal-yard and loading them onto this old truck, and carrying them on our backs into the houses. Then they had to be dumped so we'd have the sacks for the next job. I'm telling you, I ate coal dust all summer." He shook his head. "Bad enough when I got paid for my work, but let me tell you why I quit."

Chester's boss, the owner of the truck, made his living by buying coal at the coal-yard and charging enough on delivery to pay for the expenses of the truck and pay his helper, with a small profit for himself. When the coal was delivered and in the coal-bin in the basement, he went to the door for his pay. This time, the woman shook her head and said she had no money, but she needed the coal. "Come back next week," she said, shutting the door.

Enraged, for he couldn't buy another lot until he was paid for this one, the man ordered Chester to help him shovel the coal back into the sacks and carry them out to the truck, to be delivered to someone who could pay.

"Half a day wasted!" Chester said. "Then at the end of the day when he paid me he gave me 50 cents instead of a dollar, saying he couldn't afford to pay for the time at that house. I told him I couldn't afford to work for nothing, and I quit. Do you blame me?"

Old-time dances were fun, mixed with an occasional waltz or fox trot, and sometimes the lights were put out with only the stage lit for the fiddle players. That's when our partners held us closer and 'When I Grow Too Old to Dream' encouraged romantic fancies. There were box lunch nights, with decorated boxes going to the highest bidder, and costume dances.

One Saturday night Bob was taking Marshall into New Westminster after the dance as she was off the next day. I had my weekend suitcase along and they would drop me off at home for I was off too.

At one o'clock in the morning our house was dark, but I expected to find the back door unlocked. My parents knew my days off. It was locked, as were the front door and all the windows. Something about the silence of the house in spite of all my knocking told me it was empty. Bob's car was out of sight.

There was an empty lot on one side of the house, and a deaf lady lived on the other. She would never hear me. Feeling bereft, I decided to cross the street to Mrs. Plett, an elderly lady Mother had often helped when she was feeling poorly. I just wanted to be inside, safe from the menacing darkness. I would sit in a chair if necessary.

At my third knock, I heard a quavery voice ask, "Who is it?"

"It's Eva Lehman, Mrs. Plett. My parents are away and I can't get into the house."

The door opened a few inches to reveal a disapproving face and Mrs. Plett looked me up and down. "Eva! So it is! What are you doing out at this time of night?"

I explained the circumstances, saying I just wanted to be inside for the night. I didn't have to be given a bed to sleep in.

The gray old head was shaking, and Mrs. Plett's voice became strongly accusing. "Well, you can't have been up to any good, out at this hour! I knew you'd get in with bad company, out there with those nurses. Nurses! A bad lot, I say," and she closed the door firmly. I heard the key turn in the lock.

Really upset now at this unexpected condemnation and close to tears, I grasped my suitcase tightly and started off for Marshall's house. I would be on well-lighted Kingsway, the main thoroughfare between Vancouver and New Westminster, most of the way. There was a wide sidewalk and I stayed well over on the far side from the traffic. There were still cars going by, at that late hour.

A car pulled up beside me and I looked over my shoulder to see, to my intense relief, that it was a police car with two constables in the front seat. With the window down, one said, "Where are you going, young lady?"

"To the Marshalls. Four blocks from here." I had my hand on the opened window, hanging on as if to a life-line.

The policeman opened the back door. "Hop in. We'll drive you there."

I lost no time in getting into the car, and started to tell them where Marshalls lived. "I know Matt Marshall. I know where he lives," the driver said. "Are you working out at Essondale with his daughter?"

It was easy to explain what had happened, with such sympathetic listeners. I told them what Mrs. Plett had said. They looked at one another. "If we can't rouse the Marshalls I'll take you home to my wife," one of the men said.

Marshall came to the door, roused from sleep, and we waved off the police officers, whom I thanked warmly. I slept on a couch, with a blanket, and that was all I wanted. Shelter for the night. My tight-lipped mother withdrew her neighborly help to Mrs. Plett on hearing of the incident. My parents had gone out to the farm, deciding rather suddenly and forgetting that I'd be off. I should have phoned anyway, as I didn't always get home because of lectures.

I left E4 convinced it was the best place to work in the hospital. On the Admitting ward there was hope, and there was change. New patients come in, some to improve and be discharged, a lesser number to be transferred to a ward in the Chronic Building. The long-term aspect of other wards was absent, and life was much more pleasant without it.

I finished my second year of psychiatric nursing on night duty, on H3. It was uneventful except for the opportunity it gave me to become better acquainted with Hazel Groves who was on with me.

Groves was in my class but had moved out of the dormitory before I moved in so I did not know her well. She had graduated from Normal School before settling for psychiatric nursing when a school was not available. I found her to be out-going, clearly an extrovert. Efficient, obliging, cheerful, Groves was definitely headed for distinction. And so it proved.

Certainly Hazel Groves was awarded the coveted medal for general proficiency when we graduated. But more than that came her way. She kept on applying for a position as a school teacher, never expecting to be asked by Dr. Sauriol, the Superintendent of Number Nine - the former insane asylum in New Westminster - to start a school for the retarded in that institution. He had already chosen a name, The Woodlands School, and a schoolhouse with six classrooms, a Home Economics room, an Industrial Arts section, a pool and a gymnasium were on the attractive site overlooking the Fraser River.

Groves accepted with alacrity. She chose teachers, set up classes, and established a busy program for the school year. Not too many years previously, the retarded had been on the wards at Essondale with the insane. Now, the ones capable of some education and training went to school. There was never any problem with discipline at The Woodlands School. A teacher had only to say, "If you don't behave, you'll be sent back to your ward." That mild threat brought instant obedience.

A short attention span and limited abilities made a full day of classroom work impossible. Groves arranged for a one-hour period, per day, broken into 15-minute segments, for each pupil. The ward attendants collected one group of students while bringing another. All those who could walk, and some in wheelchairs, were given a chance to learn as much as they were able to assimilate. A great deal of repetition was necessary.

Besides the very basic levels of reading, writing and arithmetic, the 'children', of all ages, were trained in life situations most of them had never experienced. They learned the meaning of red and green lights at an intersection, and how to count out change - if that was possible. An increasing number of pupils progressed to the point where they were able to be placed in sheltered positions in the community. They could be seen around New Westminster buying themselves a hamburger or a doughnut, proudly counting out the correct change from money they had earned.

Groves, in true teacher fashion, had the pupils prepare for a Christmas concert to which parents and the public were invited. Two pupils importantly attended to the curtains on the stage in the gymnasium, and the clearest speaker was the master-of-ceremonies. The usual plays, drills, and songs were presented, having been rehearsed to perfection - at least as much perfection as any teacher expects at a school concert. The children loved performing and especially loved wearing costumes, made by the teachers. Songs like 'Frosty, the Snowman' meant wearing mitts and woolen caps, with a lucky pupil dressed as a snowman. They sang all the verses all the way through. Children who could not memorize otherwise learned the words of songs they loved. The level of achievement in the concert productions was astonishing, and heart-warming.

Another event arranged for the children was sports day, with a demonstration of gymnasium skills, and swimming events. Then there was Visitors' Day, with a great deal of painstaking preparation of displays of the work done in class. The Woodlands School, as set up by Hazel Groves (later Mrs. Davy), attracted continent-wide attention and served as a model for other schools for the retarded. 'Number Nine' which had previously provided purely custodial care, was now a model school.

There was no age limit in the classes. A floating teacher conducted classes on the wards, where 30 and 40-year-old spastic or otherwise disadvantaged men and women could practice school disciplines. The benefit to their morale was enormous.

The Woodlands School is situated across the street from Queen's Park in New Westminster, where a May Day festival is held every spring. Regular classes are cancelled that day so that the retarded children can see the May Queen being crowned and watch the dancing around the Maypole. A select few are taken to a reserved section of the grandstand for this ceremony, while the majority of the Woodlands residents watch the parade from the lawns on the grounds.

Mrs. Wilson, the floating teacher, was once assigned as escort to a group going to the Queen's Park grandstand for the May Day ceremonies. All six boys were strangers to her and taller than herself, and she wondered how she would be able to keep track of them. However, they walked over quietly and sat down with the other Woodlands groups to watch the games and sports. At the finish each teacher led her group out to go back to the school.

Miss Wilson was so pleased with the boys in her charge, who kept close beside her in the milling crowd of people on the grounds, that she decided to treat them to a hamburger at one of the stands. She said, as she stopped, "Wait here. I'll get you a hamburger," and went the few steps to the stall to get it.

One of the boys could not have heard her, for as she was waiting her turn, she felt a tug at her sleeve and heard his voice saying plaintively, "Teacher! You almost lost me!" Taller than herself, but still a child.

Miss Wilson had one hour a day with a bed-ridden boy who was intelligent enough to resent being in the institution. He felt rejected by his father and new mother and often spent the time he was supposed to be doing school work with the teacher, in bemoaning his fate. Before the knee operation that disabled him, he had been in a Grade Six class in a regular school and the reason for his admittance to the institution for the retarded was not clear to Miss Wilson except, perhaps, that the boy was deaf. Miss Wilson gave him directions and assigned his work by writing notes to him. Whether he would do as directed or not was another matter, as he complained bitterly every day upon her arrival at his bedside.

One day he was particularly obstreperous. Miss Wilson took the notepad and printed in large letters: READ PAGE 25 AND WRITE ANSWERS TO THE QUESTIONS. When she handed it to him, he looked at the note and said irritably, "You don't have to shout!"

The school undoubtedly brought a semblance of normalcy to many inmates of Number Nine. That name became history when the change in its goals created The Woodlands School. The educational activity that brings self-respect to pupils is a legacy from Dr. Sauriol and the psychiatric nurse and teacher, Hazel Groves Davy, commemorated in the latter case by a medal awarded in her name for proficiency in the education of the mentally disadvantaged.

CHAPTER FOURTEEN

When I came off nights I found my name on InfF, the women's infirmary. At last I would have a chance to use the techniques we had been learning in Practical Nursing. It was good to be back in the Female Chronic Building among my friends. I had been isolated too long, first on E4 and then on nights.

Gladwin and I were on the same shift again, which was great. She was worried about Don, who had lost his job at Fraser Mills and was now working in the cannery by the railway bridge in New Westminster. "But that's just summer work," Gladwin fretted. "And he has to help out at home with money. His dad was laid off too, and it's even harder for an older man to get on anywhere."

"The new bridge will be quite an improvement when it's finished," I said. "The Columbian newspaper announced that it was going to be called the Pattullo bridge, after the Premier."

"At least it will be wide enough for trucks and buses to meet. Imagine, four lanes!" The old railway bridge, planked for road traffic, had lights at each end, which the driver of a wide vehicle had to activate before he could cross. If the light was red, he had to wait for the oncoming vehicle to clear the bridge before he could start over.

"And it's high enough so the bridge doesn't have to be opened for river traffic. It's making work for construction men, too." Gladwin always came back to the lack of employment. Her young brother was out of school now and wanted work.

"Maybe next year will be better." The phrase was wearing thin, and I changed the subject. "You haven't been on InfF, Glad, have you? But you know Sullivan, the Charge Nurse. And Ferrier, and Hammond. Ferrier's on the other corridor so I won't see much of her. Which suits me fine! Hammond and I have one side each of the corridor by the office. We each have six beds with six patients to do. And they're supposed to be all bathed and their beds neat by the time Dr. Campbell makes rounds."

Hammond and I worked together, 'doing up' our patients. I felt like a true nurse at last, taking temperatures and pulse rates, handling bed-pans, and giving out medications. Miss Deroche, the Supervisor, small and dark and quick-moving, was always ready to advise and it was she who stood by when I saw my first death.

Mrs. Dease was one of my patients, and I lingered in her room more than once when the rest of my work was done, just to talk to her. She was quite weak but always responded to my chatter, seeming to take an interest in the light-hearted happenings I shared with her. I was very fond of Mrs. Dease.

Though I knew she was steadily becoming weaker, she never complained and I didn't realize she was dying. I was shocked, therefore, to walk into her room one day and find her taking shallow gasps of air, her eyes staring sightlessly at the ceiling. I ran to the office.

"Miss Deroche! Come quickly! Something's wrong with Mrs. Dease!" I expected a flurry of action but Miss Deroche calmly stood by the bed, her fingers on the sick woman's pulse. The agony of the straining breaths hurt me. I said, "Can't we do something for her?"

"She's dying," Miss Deroche informed me, her eyes on the woman's tortured face. "There's nothing we can do."

So this was Death! I stood helplessly by and felt only relief when the features relaxed and peace descended with death. Miss Deroche closed the eyelids. "I expect Dr. Campbell any minute. You can take care of the body. You've had Care of the Dead, haven't you?"

Hammond came to help me, and talked continually as we worked, understanding my distress, though the body we bathed and tended was not Mrs. Dease, as I knew her. The essence of my friend had disappeared with her death, and I couldn't mourn her passing. Not from this place.

Hammond was pulling wads of cotton batting off a roll. "The morgue attendant is furious if the body isn't prepared." she said. Hammond had been on the Infirmary a couple of months and this wasn't her first death. "So we stuff here, and here," the vagina and the anus, "because with death the sphincter muscles relax and you-know-what runs out. Not a pleasant thought, huh? Now we cross the wrists and bind them together, and the ankles. And a binder to hold the jaw closed. Not too tight, or there will be a mark when rigor mortis sets in." The body was then wrapped completely in a sheet, and lifted onto a stretcher.

An attendant arrived to take the body to the morgue, and I was told to go with him. "We always send a nurse with one of our patients," Miss Deroche said.

The attendant was an older man named Joe. He wheeled the stretcher into the elevator and we went down to one floor below the basement level. "I didn't know there was a floor below the basement," I said. "Oh, it's a tunnel!" A well-lighted passageway stretched away from us in the direction of the other buildings.

"The morgue is in the Male Chronic Building so we go all the way," Joe said. "Did you say this is the first time you're going there? Hm-m."

At the end of the tunnel we took the elevator up to the basement and went along a corridor. Joe unlocked a door, then turned to me. "Hang on for a minute while I check inside," he said, "just to make sure nobody's sitting up. Sometimes they're not quite dead when we put 'em in there." He went in and I heard loud banging, then he called, "O.K. Bring her in. I have everyone under control."

I pushed the stretcher into a large bare room, with several slabs for bodies but not a corpse in sight. Joe must have been banging a couple of head-rests around. "Trying to scare me, huh?" I laughed.

Joe became very brusque. "I'll take the head. You take the feet." We swung the body onto a slab. Joe locked the door behind us and said, "You can find your way back, I guess." He went off, and I had the eerie job of going back through the tunnel by myself.

Though I could not be sorry when a mental hospital patient died, neither could I be happy at a birth. I was present for two births while I was on InfF.

Both babies were born at night, and several nurses were called out of bed to witness the events. I hadn't been warned ahead of time, and the pregnant woman certainly hadn't been on the Infirmary ahead of time. I didn't know what to expect when Miss Marlatt wakened me, saying I was to get dressed and go over to the Infirmary.

When I arrived I was surprised to find a woman in labor with Dr. Campbell in attendance, and Miss Marlatt, Miss Hicks and Miss Deroche, and at least a dozen nurses grouped around. Hammond was one of them, and we raised our eyebrows at each other. This was better than an autopsy, anyway.

As the contractions grew more frequent, the woman's groans became agonizing. I saw Hammond make an involuntary movement toward her, almost groaning herself in sympathy. The patient moaned derisively, between gasps, "I'll have you know, nurse, that I'm the one having this baby. Not you." The sarcasm made Hammond blush.

I was able to see the miracle of the head crowning. At the next contraction the woman screamed, "Oh! I can't bear it! It's tearing me apart!" and the baby rolled out into the doctor's waiting hands. "It's a boy," he said. I wondered what would be on his birth certificate, for place of birth.

"Lehman, these will be your patients so you stay and watch me give the baby his bath, and I'll instruct you in post-partum care for Mrs. Murphy," Miss Deroche ordered. The next week was interesting and busy, as I cared for the new mother and the new-born infant.

Mrs. Murphy was quick-tempered and more concerned about her conversations with God than about her baby. When I first took the baby in to her---"Don't leave her alone with him," Miss Deroche said--- she lifted him up high and exclaimed, "The Lord picked me up and threw me down..." I hastily rescued the child, and didn't bother her with him again. She was not allowed to breast-feed him, which didn't seem to matter to her.

A crib was kept in the office and the irritable baby became the charge of anyone who was there. Miss Deroche was often found caring for him but Sullivan and Ferrier seldom looked at him. His bath and his feedings were my responsibility, but there was very little spare time to do more.

On the third day after he was born, Baby Murphy was circumcised. Dr. Campbell was attended by Miss Hicks, Miss Marlatt, and the Infirmary Supervisor. Although the baby was given a soother, a wadded sterilized bandage dipped in honey, he cried angrily, and I didn't wonder at his natural response to what I felt was an unnatural operation. "It's necessary for cleanliness," Miss Deroche told me. Really? Were men so careless with their bodies?

"They should have to menstruate every month," Dunbar said. "I wonder what they'd cut off for cleanliness then?"

The table we had appropriated as probies was still the meeting-place for our class at meals, and I was indignantly describing the circumcision I had witnessed.

"What do you think of that penis-envy theory of Freud's we had in lectures?" Renfrew asked. She scoffed, "I think it's a lot of baloney."

"It sure is," said Hammond heatedly. "Who'd want that ugly thing hanging between their legs anyway! Ugh!" She shuddered.

Oliver spoke quietly. "What would a man know about what women think? It just shows that men feel superior so they have to believe they're superior there too."

"Men are handling their penises all the time," Dunbar said with an air of authority. "Taking them out and holding them when they pee. And probably giving them a rub-up through their pants pockets. Huh!" She looked at the prune whip we were eating for dessert and announced, "None for me, thank you. Looks too much like lung tissue."

Spoons were laid down all around the table as we realized the truth of her comparison and we got up to go out on the porch for fresh air.

"But I agree," Renfrew commented on the previous topic, "A penis would be handy on a picnic."

"In more ways than one," Dunbar chuckled.

Baby Murphy was taken away by the social worker when he was ten days old, and Mrs. Murphy was returned to her ward. She never asked about the child she'd borne with so much suffering. "He threw me down three times before I accepted His word," she chanted.

The second birth I witnessed was much easier. There was no sound from the mother during labor. She was a contented, placid woman, and her contented baby slept between feedings and never cried. The mother was totally inept in regard to the baby and was happy to leave his care to the nurses. When he was taken away by the social worker she didn't care, or ask about him.

"Whoever said everyone was born equal was away off track," was Oliver's conclusion. We all agreed.

There were two corridors on InfF and six rooms on each side of each corridor. Though Ferrier was Sullivan's friend, she was assigned the side that had the 'shit woman' in the end room. Very little could be done for this unfortunate woman. She rubbed her own excrement all over herself and streaked it down the walls. She ate it. Her teeth were plugged with it and her hair stood out in stiff strands where she had run her shitty hands through and through. Her fingernails were filthy. She stank.

Ferrier slid a tray in for each meal, and shut the door fast, for the deranged woman delighted in smearing other people. Rubber gloves had to be worn picking up the tray at the door, for it was smeared with feces and had to be put into an antiseptic solution and scrubbed with a brush. A set of trays was reserved for this patient, and her food transferred to them at meal times.

Every so often--not every day---she was cleaned up. The first time I helped with this, I was not prepared for the apparition we were approaching, but I soon found that her arms had to be held, and held tightly, for she was wiggly as an eel and her shit-filled hands were gleefully drawn down the nurses' arms before we knew it. While the nurses stripped off her brown-streaked nightgown and put her under the shower, a cleaning woman was busy with soapsuds washing off the bedstead, the walls, and the floor. The smell was over-powering.

The worst of the filthy job was knowing it was useless. She would have herself and her room covered with shit as soon as she could produce it again.

Being sent downstairs to the basement laboratory for autopsy viewing was still a part of our nursing education. While I was on the Women's Infirmary I went down and found Miss Marlatt wearing a gown and rubber gloves, scalpel in hand, performing the post-mortem examination of a body. Dr. Byrne, who appeared uncomfortable as a spectator, stood with Miss Hicks nearby, and the usual complement of nurses had come in to observe. The surprise on everyone's face showed that no one had been told that gentle Miss Marlatt would be wielding the knife. Somehow I received the impression that this was the result of a dare, or a taunt about the abilities of a woman, for when all was done, Dr. Byrne moved as if to take over, saying, "That's enough, now. I'll finish up." Miss Marlatt stood firm. "No. I'll do the sewing too," and she did, to the last stitch.

The girls filed out at a signal from Miss Hicks, and there was an air of jubilation amongst us that supported my idea of it being a test of the competence of women. Miss Hicks had chosen well for her Assistant Superintendent of Nurses. Miss Marlatt looked fragile, but she had a core of steel.

Now we were third year students. Seniors. I had gone on nights just in time to miss this year's graduation exercises, for I was on duty. Next year would be ours. One more year of lectures. I hoped there would be a job, somewhere else, not so isolated.

I was in uniform early one afternoon making myself some tea in the kitchen of the Home. I had put the kettle on when Miss Hicks came in. She spoke in her brisk way, "Miss Lehman, you have plenty of time before you go on duty. Will you make up a tray for Miss Marlatt, please? Just tea and toast. No, nothing else. Thank you. Bring it up to our suite as soon as it's ready." Again I had been caught for an unusual task. Miss Marlatt must be ill.

I found a cloth for the tray and set out a cup and saucer, cream and sugar, and a plate for the toast which was almost ready. The kettle was boiling, so I made tea in one small pot and filled another with hot water. With the buttered toast on the plate, I picked up the tray and went up the stairs to their door.

Miss Hicks thanked me and said she would return everything to the kitchen. Miss Marlatt did not come back on duty, and we heard eventually that she was in the TB sanitorium in Tranquille. She did not conquer the disease. Tuberculosis claimed a fine, gentle nurse, much admired and mourned by the student body.

A startling revelation eventually resulted in my complicity in deception.

"I guess you haven't heard Dunbar's latest," Gladwin had said to me a month before. "She's bragging about her week-ends at a beach-house in White Rock. The way she tells it, there's three couples and two double beds, so they draw straws to see which couple gets a bed to themselves. Do you believe it?"

"From what I've been hearing from Sullivan and Ferrier I'd say it could be true, Gladdie. How do you suppose they keep from getting pregnant?" Neither of us knew.

Later I was on night duty with Dunbar, on ward J. We were walking back to the Home one morning, four of us, all from our class. Hammond and Oliver were on nights, too, and we had met for breakfast. We listened to Dunbar's outrageous chatter thinking that she was surely stretching the truth in her desire to appear sophisticated. She just wanted to shock us.

All at once Dunbar turned aside and vomited onto the grass beside the walk. The three of us exchanged startled looks and waited for her, as she wiped her mouth. Nonchalantly, almost proudly, Dunbar said, "I was wondering whether I'd get morning sickness in the morning or when I got up in the afternoons. Isn't that interesting! I really thought it'd be in the afternoons, being we're on nights." Her insouciance amazed us, and we were silent as we went into the Home. What would be a disaster to us didn't seem to bother her at all.

A few nights later Dunbar had news for me. "I went to the doctor today. He gave me some pills that might take effect tonight or tomorrow. I hope they work. If I'm not here tomorrow you'll know they worked. The doctor said I'd only miss a couple of shifts."

"What will you say when Miss Windermere asks why you were off?" I asked in fascination. It was hard to believe this girl, so pretty and with such an innocent-looking face, could be in this predicament. I was more troubled than she appeared to be.

"The doctor said he'd phone with some excuse. I suppose I could have a broken arm."

"Dunbar! If you say you have broken your arm, you'd have to have it in a cast for weeks! Think of something else."

Dunbar suggested the flu. I was doubtful, but I had an idea. "No, if you have the flu you'd have to stay away longer than two nights, or be awfully weak when you get back. How about ptomaine poisoning? It doesn't last long if you get to a doctor. We'd better look up the symptoms so you can tell Windermere when you're back. She's sure to ask."

Dunbar lasted the night, though saying she was getting an occasional cramp by morning. I was not surprised at her absence the next two nights. The relief nurse took her place and Miss Windermere informed me, "Miss Dunbar is off with ptomaine poisoning. Her doctor phoned. I guess she's pretty sick."

Dunbar came back, pale and languid. "That was tougher than I thought it would be," she said wanly.

The Night Supervisor was impressed by Dunbar's pale face, in marked contrast to her usual rosy glow. "You've had a tough time," she sympathized. I kept my eyes on the floor, afraid I would reveal Dunbar's deceit by the expression on my face. Miss Windermere went on, "How bad were your symptoms? What do you suppose caused it?"

The corner of her mouth twitching, Dunbar told about her cramps, and added, "And terrible diarrhea and vomiting, until the medicine the doctor gave me took effect. I emptied out everything that was in my stomach." The minx was enjoying this!

"What do you think you ate?" Miss Windermere asked. "It wouldn't be the meals here; nobody else has had poisoning."

"I think it was what I had in White Rock," Dunbar said. "I was there for the weekend."

"You have to watch what you eat at those beach resorts," the Supervisor warned, and left us to dissolve into giggles as soon as we heard the door clang shut behind her.

On Dunbar's nights off, I was in charge of Ward J, for the relief nurse was junior to me. We always worked together, so the biggest difference to me was having to write up the report for the day staff's information. Making the rounds with McKenzie, the Charge Nurse on days, was easy as everyone was securely locked into separate side-rooms so the count was more of a check on each room.

When the two night nurses had taken each patient to the washroom in turn, there was little to do until the doctor made his visit. He ordered a sedative injection or paraldehyde for women whose noise was disturbing the ward. Though giving a hypodermic needle to a squirming, unco-operative patient was dangerous---my worry was that the needle would break and be imbedded in her flesh, as I had heard could happen---I preferred that method to giving paraldehyde, a viscous liquid with an overpoweringly disagreeable smell.

The medicine must have tasted as bad as it smelled for invariably the woman spit it back at us. While one of us held her as tightly as possible, the other closed the woman's nostrils with one hand and held the medicine glass to her mouth with the other when the unfortunate woman gasped for air. It was a barbaric procedure and coming away from it with the vile smell of paraldehyde on our uniforms, to be with us the rest of the night, seemed fitting punishment for having inflicted it on the patient, although we had not ordered it. We wondered if the doctors had ever smelled paraldehyde, or given it. Not likely.

With the drugs administered and the ward quieted down, we had the rest of the long night to ourselves, with one break for the midnight meal. We sat at the big desk in the office, which was at the end of one of the two corridors of rooms. Dunbar and I were able to study together, having the same lectures. We checked our notes for accuracy and completeness, and quizzed each other for exams. We both were avid readers, and I even taught her to knit, passing along the skills Mrs. Cook had taught me on F3.

It was also pleasant working with the relief nurse, Heffley, who was energetic and high-spirited. We worked well together.

Heffley was with me one night when paraldehyde was ordered for a very noisy patient. "Let me measure that out," Heffley said while I was preparing syringes for injections. I knew by her tone that she was going to compensate for the amount usually spit out so that the woman would cease her yelling, but a glance at the glass showed very little over the mark and I let it go. The ward was soon quiet and the night passed peacefully.

In the morning when we came to her room, almost the last one to do, the paraldehyde patient was snoring loudly, dead to the world. Something about the ragged breathing alarmed us. Heffley looked as stricken as I felt, as we remembered the extra bit of medicine. Regardless of who measured it out, it was my responsibility.

We dragged her to her feet and into the bathroom, where we put her into a cold shower. We alternated the shower and walking her up and down, but she was still groggy and unsteady when the day staff came on duty. I read the report with a leaden heart, not yet confessing that an overdose, however small, had been given. Our guilty consciences made Heffley and me believe we had almost finished the woman.

The Charge Nurse's reaction to the report was surprising. McKenzie was large, solid and unflappable, but when I read, 'Paraldehyde to the patient in room 14' she interrupted, 'Paraldehyde! Did that woman get paraldehyde?' I nodded, and miserably told her of the woman's condition and our efforts to revive her. Heffley was still with her in the washroom.

Before I could go on to reveal the overly-generous measure which Heffley and I believed was responsible for the frightening stupor the woman was in, and which we bitterly regretted, McKenzie, to my complete astonishment said, "We'll take over now. You've been doing exactly the right things. I'm sure she'll be fine when you come on tonight." I closed my mouth and thankfully made the count, then departed with a subdued Heffley.

"Gosh, Lehman, I'm sure sorry," she started on an apology as we went down the stairs. "I don't care how much they spit back, I'll never measure out a smidgen more than the right dose from now on. I was never so scared...!"

"Me too," I agreed. "But wasn't it queer that McKenzie took it so quietly! She almost looked scared too. I was sure we were in for it; in fact I wouldn't have been surprised to be sent down to Miss Hick's office. I even imagined we'd both be fired."

When we came on duty that evening, we found all serene. The paraldehyde patient looked fully recovered, and McKenzie told me on rounds her part in the nearly fatal incident.

"I was plenty scared," she confessed. "That woman had a sedative after the doctor's rounds in the morning, and she was still kicking up holy hell hours later. So we fixed her up a pill sandwich, off the record, to get some peace on the ward. And she was still making a racket at ten o'clock at night? No wonder you asked for sedation for her! Then I guess the whole thing hit her all at once. I don't know why I consented to the pill sandwich. We were at our wit's end. But it's my responsibility and my say-so. I'll tell you one thing:

I'll put up with any amount of noise from now on rather than have that happen again. You kids must have been scared out of your minds."

"What's a pill sandwich?" Heffley asked when we were alone and I had related the day staff's involvement in the mishap, to her great relief.

"I've never heard of it before," I said. "But I would guess it's a way of getting a patient to take a pill, putting it in a jam or peanut butter sandwich. We don't seem to get orders for pills at night, I guess because there's only two of us and the patients aren't that co-operative. Well, we were lucky on that one. I don't actually think that overdose had very much to do with her passing out, but we won't take the chance again, I'll bet." Heffley fervently agreed.

The most valuable lessons that I learned as a psychiatric nurse were the revelations of human nature and behavior. For three years packed with incongruous experiences I lived and worked with young women from many backgrounds, with differing standards and morals. We shared happiness and suffering, fear and courage, laughter and tears. We depended on one another in potentially dangerous circumstances. We talked and shared confidences. We faced enmity and aggression together. We grew very close, and life-long friendships developed.

Young nurses were taken in hand by those whose special characteristics had earned them positions as Charge or Supervisor, and by special people like my friend Marshall who included us in her activities and amusements. In retrospect I concluded that there were more pluses than minuses to being a psychiatric nurse.

CHAPTER FIFTEEN

Since meeting the young men in the neighborhood at the weekly dances through the winters, we had become interested in their football games. Football had been a favorite spectator sport in High School, but it was not football as it is known today. The ball was propelled mainly by kicking, as in the game called soccer now.

Several communities in the valley had teams and there was keen rivalry between Port Coquitlam, Mission, Kilgard, Abbotsford, and Langley. Clubs were formed and money was raised to buy the players shorts and sweaters by holding dances, whist drives, crib games, and raffles. As well, a hat was passed around at games which were otherwise free. My friends and I were included in as many of these activities as our time off allowed.

Hammond, Marshall and I had been the most regular dancers and this was our third winter with the group. So when Chester presented us with a venison roast, the parcel that arrived at the Nurses' Home was addressed to the three of us.

"There's a present for you, Lehman," Keith informed me when I came off duty. "A very polite young man asked me to put it in the fridge. It's for Hammond and Marshall too." Her eyes were twinkling. "A taste of deer for tasteful dears," the note read. What a strange gift!

We didn't know much about cooking a roast, so we consulted Keith. She advised us to make a paste of flour and water to put on it, "to keep the juices in," and also suggested the temperature and the time to cook it. We promptly invited her to eat with us later. It was a large roast so we asked Oliver and Gladwin, and Miss Whitehorse.

After all, we were monopolizing her kitchen and also, we wanted to use some of the vegetables that were on hand for her suppers. Although we had eaten three meals that day, the venison was delicious. Miss Whitehorse didn't scold us for not being finished before the hour we were supposed to be in our rooms. She even smiled once or twice at our light-hearted banter.

Hammond and I composed a letter of thanks to Chester, praising him for his prowess with a rifle and for his generosity in sharing the venison with us. Marshall signed it too, and we made a great ceremony out of presenting it to him at the next dance. It was a rare, unexpected treat. We didn't have much money, but we made our own fun.

Lectures in our third year were tough. Drugs and Solutions. Pathology. Communicable and Infectious Diseases. Obstetrics, and, of course, Psychiatry, specifically the findings of Freud, Jung, Adler.

We were given the theories of psychoanalysis, dream interpretation and the use of hypnosis in the treatment of the mentally ill, but were not told whether they were used by the doctors at Essondale, or not. Nurses were not encouraged to participate in the treatment of patients except in a subservient role, such as handing the doctor the instruments he needed.

On the Men's Infirmary, my next placement, much of the bedside nursing was done by male attendants. Four nurses and four attendants staffed E2, the men taking care of bedbaths, bedpans, and enemas. The nurses took temperatures and recorded other vital signs, gave out medications, sanitized equipment and rolled bandages. When a procedure such as a lumbar puncture was underway, I might be present, though the ward Supervisor, Miss Ashcroft, was always at the doctor's right hand. She was the equivalent of the scrub nurse at an operation, and I was the float. The gopher. "Go for this," and "Go for that." Actually, our medical trays were meticulously made up and there was little for me to do but watch.

The other two nurses were Ella Lord and Bradner, the Charge. Bradner was very particular about the care of the patients and the appearance of the ward, and it seemed she could always find something for her nurses to do.

I had been on ward E2 for a couple of weeks, when one of the attendants decided to cut down on my work. "What are you rushing about for, now?" he would ask. "Do you have to?" Hamilton was a fatherly type, the Head Attendant. The men took a much more leisurely view of their job than the nurses though they were accountable to Miss Ashcroft and Bradner. They were quite adept at appearing to be busy, and they lightened their days from time to time with practical jokes, which in some instances turned out to be anything but funny.

"Come on," Hamilton was saying now. "We need a fourth at bridge. You girls run around like chickens with their heads cut off. Miss Bradner wants you to roll bandages? Well, roll a couple and then come and join us."

I did play bridge occasionally on E2, with a deaf-mute patient and two attendants. "Hurry up, Lehman, and sit down here. Smiley needs to be amused and if we can get started you're doing a favor for a patient, see?"

Playing bridge with the deaf-mute involved some interesting hand signals and required unflagging attention. The number of tricks bid was shown first by holding up that number of fingers. Spades were indicated by a digging motion, hearts by touching one hand to your breast. Clubs were a shake of the fist, and diamonds were shown by touching the third finger of the left hand, the ring finger. No trump was a finger on the lips, pass was a slap on the table. Smiley was a good bridge player, and the men made sure he was amused practically every afternoon.

The casual attitude of the attendants relieved many a situation that would otherwise have been depressing. There was the incident of the pipe-smoker, which was typical of their sense of humor. A patient had died, the doctor had verified the death, and Miss Ashcroft asked Hamilton and Burns to prepare the body for the morgue.

"Let's have some excitement around here," urged Burns, in a devilish mood. They propped the corpse up on his pillows, put his pipe in his mouth, and put on a great show. "Miss Ashcroft! Come quick! Old Powell isn't dead. He's sitting up smoking his pipe!"

Three of us hurried down to Powell's room, to discern the charade immediately. "Oh, you guys!" Miss Ashcroft said good-humoredly. "Come on! We have better things to do than put up with your nonsense."

The attendants played jokes on each other, too. Sometimes they were unwittingly cruel, as when Creston, new on the job, was sent over to the morgue when a call came from the Female Chronic Building for an attendant to accompany a nurse with a body.

"Here's a chance for you to meet one of the nurses, Creston. Who knows, she may be pretty, not like the ones on this ward," with a sideways glance at me. I was used to their teasing by now.

They told Creston where the morgue was, and to ask at the Information Desk in the Female Chronic Building for the Infirmary, where he would pick up the body. "Good luck," they chuckled. They neglected to tell him about the tunnel connecting the buildings.

The accompanying nurse had evidently never been through the tunnel either, for Creston pushed the stretcher through uncleared snow from the Female Building to the Male Building, and like the gentleman he was, he pushed the empty stretcher back for the pretty nurse. By the time he returned to E2 he was ruddy with cold, and ready to sit down and rest. Miss Ashcroft, who knew nothing about the practical joke, met him as soon as he came onto the ward. "Oh, Creston. I've had a phone call from the Charge Nurse, and that body wasn't supposed to go to the morgue. It's going straight to the lab for an autopsy. So you're to go and pick it up at the morgue and take it back to the Female Chronic Building."

When Creston came back after his second trip, he was exhausted. "Three times I pushed that damn stretcher between those buildings," he said angrily. "Dumb clucks, anyway, sending for me to take a body to the morgue when it was supposed to go for an autopsy." His remarks about the intelligence of women were scathing.

Burns and Hamilton looked at one another, and suddenly found something to do for the sick patients. When Creston found out about the tunnel, they hoped he would have been moved to another ward. Their practical joke had gone farther than they intended.

Gladwin and I were having our end-of-the-day exchange of news. I told her about Creston's trips in the snow, and added, "Ward E2 is fine, less work than on the Female Infirmary, but I miss seeing everyone at meals and getting the latest gossip. What's new?"

We discussed her constant worry, Don, who was now unemployed for the winter. "His dad's on relief," Gladwin said. "And that doesn't make him very happy. That new pension plan that has come in isn't paid out until you're 70. Don's dad has 20 years yet."

To lighten her mood I started talking about a young doctor who was taking his internship in psychiatry and had been on E2 for part of that day. Ella Lord had been passing Dr. Ryan's office when Dr. Lougheed first came, and in the way the Medical staff had of asking any available nurse to run errands for them, Dr. Ryan asked Lord to show the new doctor to his office. "The second door around the corner," he explained.

Of course he had not taken the utility room into consideration, so Lord led Dr. Lougheed around the corner and opened the second door, to the sight of mops and cleaning supplies and a deep sink in a tiny room. "I could have sunk through the floor," Lord said, her face screwed up into a knot. But she laughed with us when she described it later at the table.

Dr. Lougheed was undoubtedly brainy, so deep in his own thoughts that he often appeared unaware of his surroundings. The story went around that he went out the stairway door to go down a floor, and then forgot about the stairs and fell down the cement steps. If it was true, he wasn't hurt enough for it to show.

And now Miss Hicks was receiving a gentleman caller! I was near the front door one evening when the doorbell rang, and I answered it. A tall man, older than any that ever called on the nurses, asked for Miss Hicks. He was wearing a blue three-piece suit with a tie, and he carried a hat in his hand. Not our casual young men at all.

I showed him into the lounge, thinking, "I can't stand at the bottom of the stairs and holler, "Miss Hicks!" I went up and knocked at her door, and saw that she was expecting her visitor. "Tell him I'll be down right away," she said, her color high. I wasted no time in passing the word around and soon we all knew that Miss Hicks was being courted.

Miss Hicks became Mrs. Ben Lang the following year, and of course she left her position at Essondale to become a wife and mother, living in New Westminster. It was there that our paths crossed again many years later, when our children were going to the same school and Mrs. Lang and I both worked for the PTA. I would never have dreamed when I was taking her training course that one day I would walk into her home and she would visit mine, while planning a PTA bazaar. "I'm going to write about my three years at Essondale some day," I told her. "Do you mind if I use your name?"

"Not at all," she answered in her brisk way. "Let me know when you get it done."

When the Langs moved to Victoria shortly afterward, I lost touch with her. The only word I had was that she had died of cancer at an early age. I remember Miss Hicks with gratitude and admiration. Every young person needs a model, someone who represents the kind of person he or she would like to be. Unlikely as it was that I could ever be as capable and kind as Miss Hicks, she was the epitome of excellence to me.

Fourteen of our class graduated as full-fledged psychiatric nurses. Renfrew, who had repeated a year of high school and was not a high school graduate when she started, though she ostensibly had '4th year' when we applied, had to repeat her third year of lectures. Groves received the general proficiency award, and went on to become Principal of the Woodlands School. She was liked by everybody, and we all approved her award.

For the third year Oliver achieved the highest marks, and her parents were there to see their ramrod-straight daughter go up to receive her prize. Oliver was going to leave at the end of July, to go into a five-year course in Nursing Administration at the University of British Columbia. She told me she used her psychiatry notes from Essondale as a basis for her fifth-year thesis and got Honors standing on it. She earned two degrees in that course, Bachelor of Science, and Registered Nurse, having written R.N. exams along the way.

Predictably, Oliver became a Superintendent of Nurses, a very good one. Her nursing students had a superior model in Miss Oliver, but it is doubtful if any of them could emulate her upright bearing.

I was planning to be married in June, so I would be working only one month after graduation. I had met Douglas at the New Westminster Library only six months before.

I had been following him out of the library with my arms full of books, as his were, and he held the door open for me. One of my books slipped out of the pile, we bent down at the same time to retrieve it, and our heads bumped together. Perhaps the stars we saw had something to do with the instant attraction felt by both of us.

He was apologizing and I was thanking him, for he had picked up the book first, when he exclaimed, "You're not going to carry all those books, are you? How far do you have to go? Three miles! Oh no, I'll drive you home."

On that short trip we discovered much about each other. Doug was reading The Forsyte Saga and I was familiar with Galsworthy's novels. I had found the third book in the Jalna series and started him reading Mazo de la Roche.

Douglas was 26, and he batched with his dad since his mother had died two years earlier. He had fairly steady work at a paper mill, where he had been since high school. His ten-year old Chev was so well cared for that it looked like new. "My friends say you could eat your lunch off the engine," he said with some pride. "An engine runs better if it's clean, I tell them." He was ready for marriage. "Just waiting to meet the right girl," he said fondly.

A friend of our family offered to make my wedding dress as a wedding present, if I would buy the material. Satin for a full slip and lace for the dress cost nearly ten dollars.

Gladwin was my maid-of-honor and she bought a floor-length rose satin dress with a pleated bodice and a full skirt, for six dollars. The color suited her dark hair and outdoorsy complexion which she had retained in spite of all our night duty.

For our honeymoon we drove to the Okanagan, the first time for either of us. The Fraser Canyon road was dirt and gravel surfaced, and so narrow in places that meeting a car meant going dangerously close to the unprotected edge, with the river far below. Where there are tunnels today the road went out around the mountainside, and where bridges span a ravine, we drove all the way in to the narrowest place for a bridge, and all the way back on the other side.

Looking ahead in places such as the approach to the old Alexandra Bridge, we saw the road built out on wooden supports around some of the corners. The road had been changed very little since it was constructed by the Royal Engineers for the Gold Rush, to transport supplies to the camps and ore to the ships on the Coast.

Without credit cards everyone paid cash. Our five day trip, for gas, hotels, and meals, cost $75. Traffic was light, and most cars on the road were relics of the Depression, older than ours. We came back to live with Doug's dad, taking over the expenses of the house, and lucky to have a place to live. We were the first of our age group to be married, for boys in their 20s did not often have the means to support a wife and family.

A couple of years later I was invited by Oliver - she was living with her parents - to a bridal shower for Hammond, and there we caught up on everyone's news. We reminisced about the dormitory and Miss Whitehorse with her suspicious nature. "She can't still be alive," Gladwin said.

"Oh, but she is," Oliver claimed. "She's in a nursing home in North Vancouver. Probably telling everyone they mustn't sleep together."

We were all agog about Hammond's romance and her plans for marriage. She was marrying a Mountie, and would live in Frobisher Bay. "Frobisher Bay!" we chimed. "Isn't that in the Arctic?"

Larry was in Frobisher Bay, on Baffin Island, and would be flying back for the wedding. "He wrote to tell me what clothes I would need for the Arctic," Hammond laughed. "He said I absolutely had to have long-johns. Do you know the stores don't carry long underwear for women any more? So there I was, in the men's department, having to choose between a drop seat or a pull apart style. The front arrangement isn't so handy, either."

Under cover of the laughter Hammond said to me in a low voice, "I've never thanked you Lehman, for listening to me and putting your arms around me when I told you my troubles. I think I expected that you'd despise me..."

"Never!" I interrupted. "Just because your father took advantage of you with his authority as a father! Who would blame you?" I hugged her again, happy that she had found happiness.

Marshall was at the shower, too. She and Bob were not married yet, and she was still working at Essondale. They didn't marry until he joined the Air Force when the war started. He applied for pilot's training and passed the examinations, realizing an ardent ambition.

Before he could be sent overseas he developed an eye infection which left him with less than 20-20 vision, and he was discharged as unfit for war service. He moped around home for a time, then heard that pilots were needed in South America, and he went there. With a job as a commercial pilot, he wanted the family - there were three children - to move to Peru.

Marshall refused, Bob went anyway without her, and the years went by until Bob retired, and he came back, to stay.

Marshall's sacrifice to Bob's selfishness in going his way, leaving her to raise three children and work to support them - for we saw no more sign of financial than of moral support from Bob - was incredible. In all the years until he retired, he was home only twice, and he seemed to think Marshall should join him in Peru with the children. Maybe she should have. But she wanted the children to go to school here and speak English, and she had work she liked. By now she was a Charge Nurse at Essondale with better pay. Bob's sister had moved in with her and looked after the children, who, understandably, would have nothing to do with their father when he did come home.

What really startled us, though, was that when Bob came back to retire he moved in with Marshall and she was pleased as punch to have him back. The children were married and away. His sister was no longer part of the household. "It beats me," said Gladwin. "I'd never forgive him. Lord knows what he was up to all those years in South America."

Gladwin had not married. When the war started in 1939 Don was one of the first to join up, as he hadn't held a steady job ever - Fraser Mills was only part time work. Glad's brother joined up, too. It wasn't patriotism that led to their decision, it was the chance to have decent clothes and regular meals and money in their pockets.

They were both killed overseas. Gladwin lost her father, her brother and the man she loved, in wars. She left Essondale to work at Royal Columbian Hospital as an aide, so she could live at home and support her aging mother, who was worn out from a lifetime of hard work. She, too, had lost her husband and her son, and the chance of having grandchildren.

Marshall kept us informed of changes at the mental hospital. It was a sad day when she told us what happened to Keith, the Charge who watched over her nurses and protected them from the pitfalls of living with all types of individuals.

After years of service devoted to the welfare of her patients and her staff on ward F4, and to the maintenance of the ward itself in as nearly new condition as could be managed, Keith was rewarded with an appointment as Day Supervisor of the Nurses' Home. She was an excellent choice for the position as she was well-liked. She herself was ecstatic.

For three years the Home and the girls thrived under Keith's caring ministrations. Then one day she made a fateful decision. In the supply cupboard was an almost full can of floor wax which had become cracked and dry, unfit for use.

Keith had lived through a ten-year economic depression, and she had been brought up to waste not, want not. She decided to soften the wax in the oven.

How long she left it there we don't know. When she opened the oven door the tin exploded in flames. Keith grabbed oven mitts and carried the burning wax out of the kitchen door, with the flames blowing back onto her face, her hair, and her uniform. She threw the can ahead of her and ran screaming from the building, in flames from head to foot.

A man working near by reached her first and wrapped her in his coat, then rolled her on the ground to put out the flames. She was taken to a hospital, but she lived only three days. Then, mercifully, she died.

A medal is presented each year to the best psychiatric nurse in the graduating class in memory of Miss Keith, that exceptional person who died protecting her beloved Home and fellow nurses from the holocaust of fire, and suffered it herself. The nurses who receive the Annie S. Keith Award, offered by the Psychiatric Nurses' Association, are not as fortunate as those of us who knew and worked with Annie Keith.

Many changes have taken place since my three years at the Provincial Mental Hospital at Essondale during the Depression in the 1930's, and more changes are proposed at this writing. Riverview, as the hospital complex was renamed, was affected by many factors that created new situations calling for new solutions. The search for the perfect answer to the problems of mental illness continues. Mental Health has to be of interest to all humankind.

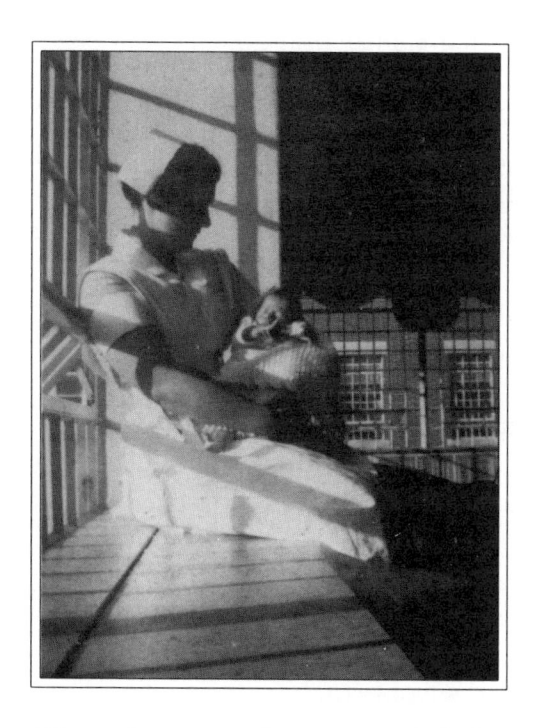

The author cares for a patient's baby.

CHAPTER SIXTEEN

Active treatment of the mentally ill began shortly after I gave up my work as a psychiatric nurse. In the late 1930's patients were given insulin shock with some beneficial results, and the procedure became a daily occurrence. Electroconvulsive therapy followed and replaced insulin shock to a large extent. Electric shock is still in use today though more discrimination is employed in selecting suitable recipients than when the method was in the experimental stages. Metrazol, a new drug, was efficacious as a circulatory and respiratory stimulant in shock therapy.

The war years, 1939-1946, brought new problems of space and staffing. Patient numbers were steadily increasing due to a fast-growing population, people from other parts of Canada being attracted by the milder climate of the West Coast, and to longer life spans resulting from improvements in health care.

Male and female staff members left to join the armed forces or to take better paying jobs now being offered. From having their pick from the large number of unemployed, the Administration now was faced with a shortage of help.

The return of married graduates such as Marshall alleviated the situation somewhat but the turnover among student nurses accelerated to the point where the average length of stay was less than one year. Experienced staff were overburdened by the larger numbers of patients - wards that formerly accommodated 100 now squeezed in half as many again - and there was a shortage of recruits to compensate for the situation.

Somehow the training program was continued. At the request of three male attendants they were allowed to take the lecture course and graduate as psychiatric nurses. By 1942 nine men had completed the training, and the number swelled to 26 in l946. A separate course for male attendants was then set up and formerly custodial and disciplinary care was replaced by the professional knowledge of trained, informed employees.

In l948 a group of sorely-pressed nurses presented the Administration with a list of suggestions for improvements in their working conditions. These were acted upon and many benefits resulted.

The first request was for the introduction of eight-hour shifts to attract more staff. This was done. More and more Nurses' Homes had to be built, one a four-storied building, and they numbered from Nurses' Home No. l to No. l0, an indication of the tremendous increase in the number of patients that had taken place.

A recreational hall was built for the use of patients and staff. Now there was a dance floor, a canteen, and a gymnasium. No longer did a ward dayroom have to be cleared for graduation exercises. The increase in leisure time that accompanied shorter working hours could be spent profitably in healthy pursuits in Pennington Hall.

Senile patients had been moved to buildings vacated by the Boys' Industrial School, when it was moved elsewhere. More buildings were constructed for male and female senile patients on those grounds as their numbers increased, and more staff had to be employed.

Bus service was improved and a bus station was built, also a canteen. Buildings sprang up for the Provincial Mental Hospital Employees Association's Credit Union and a bank. An Education building and a Nurses' Infirmary were built.

A major change that was made following the nurses' petition was that support staff were hired to relieve patients and nurses from cleaning and housekeeping duties, and from kitchen and dining room work. Marshall did not think this was all to the good. "The workers used to have a change from the dayroom," she said. "Now the days stretch out emptily and all they have to occupy themselves with are the OT for some, and an occasional movie or a dance. The routine was good for them. If it was felt the work should be paid for, why not pay the patients who wanted to do it?"

All of the auxiliary services had to be increased and more space provided. With attic and basement wards being opened, the facilities formerly quartered there were moved to new buildings, one for

Supplies, one for the Bakery, one for the Laundry, and others. The hillside became dotted with buildings.

The new Laundry that opened in 1941 had to be enlarged in 1947. A Laundry report for the year 1947 serves as an example of the work created by the rapid expansion.

In that year it was estimated that 1,737,025 pounds of articles needing washing passed through the machines in the Essondale Laundry. The washers, dryers and presses handled 650,000 sheets; 25,000 blankets; 120,000 nurses' uniform pieces: bibs, caps, dresses, aprons, collars, cuffs and belts; doctors' white coats; towels, tablecloths, kitchen aprons; bakery workers' aprons and high white hats; patients' clothes and ward clothing: dresses, slips, nightgowns, men's pants and shirts, underwear; bedspreads, pillow cases.

Every three weeks it was necessary to make 5000 pounds of germicidal soap to be used in the Laundry. Five miles of tape were used for marking items every year.

Though support staff was hired in other areas of the hospital, the Laundry continued to use patients, male and eventually female helpers. The operation of laundry equipment was considered a useful skill in obtaining work upon discharge.

Besides the three large buildings lined up on the hillside which were in use when I was a psychiatric nurse, a fourth brick building stood vacant all through the Depression and the war years. Known as the Veterans' building, it had been intended to accommodate soldiers returned from the War of 1914-1918 in a disturbed mental state. Lack of money to furnish and operate it were the reasons it was not used until it was opened as the Crease Clinic in time to treat disoriented civilian and military victims of Hitler's war.

Now the Crease Clinic, after 50 years of service, is being vacated again because of de-institutionalization. The Male Chronic Building (renamed West Lawn), the oldest of the three on the hill is empty of patients. Movie crews use it when an institutional building such as a jail is required for shooting. The other two, now called Center Lawn and East Lawn, are still in use and will likely remain so for some years to come. Though modern drugs and treatments have released many formerly mentally ill people to normal life, a core of patients remain who do not respond favorably to the methods in use.

It must be said that normal life has changed for everyone with the advent of mental hospital patients in the community. The police forces and health services are overburdened with cases which did not exist, or very rarely existed, before medicines such as Chlorpromazine changed excitable, agitated persons into tranquil, amenable citizens - if they take the medicine as prescribed, and if the dosage is correct at each stage of their behavior problem. Now the bag ladies and vagrant men are out on the streets, and whether they are better off than in an institution is debatable. Conditions in some of the substitute homes, or the halfway houses, are often proved to be vastly inferior to those in the mental hospital. The cost of the institution has been shifted to the social services and the health system, and to policing and prisons.

The large, overcrowded state hospitals as I knew them provided protection and custody, but little therapy. Patients were under benevolent surveillance by friendly nurses who treated them with kind firmness and matter-of-fact acceptance. Those who were naked were given sedatives and clothed. Aggressiveness was controlled, destructive impulses curbed.

Families were relieved of the care and responsibility that was a threat to their own health. The family today which has had a member returned to its care finds normal life disrupted to the point of despair. Suicidal threats may lead to continual fear, a state of anxiety that is detrimental to the health of the rest of the family. Mental and physical exhaustion sets in for the caregiver, with feelings of shame, or guilt, and often hurt from the criticisms of others. They are faced with the financial drain of medicines and treatments; there may be expensive psychoanalysis. Taxpayers are not released from the costs of mental illness with the closure of mental hospitals. They now shoulder costs of public assistance programs; mental health centers, doctors, nurses, counsellors and rehabilitation workers dealing with the problem.

Ordinary community members are not exempt from the consequences of empty mental hospitals. They face greater risks, with news reports revealing increasing violence and rape. Children must be taught to be suspicious of strangers. They are exposed to the temptations of mood-altering drugs at an early age. Where is the carefree childhood of 50 years ago?

Antipsychotic drugs which made de-institutionalization possible are not considered desirable by some of the disturbed individuals who have been subjected to their effects. In spite of favorable reports from attending physicians who felt the drugs had been beneficial, two mentally unstable persons made their feelings known in these accounts:

'Believe me, after spending ten months as an involuntary mental patient in Riverview, followed by two consecutive years to date in a mental health boarding home ... I know that psychotropic drugs are definitely not the answer.

'Just as religious fanatics have a right to pattern their lifestyles according to their precious delusions, without being considered victims of some supposed biochemical imbalance, so I believe that I should be free to live according to my own fantasies, without being forced to suffer the debilitating side effects of the psychiatric drugs...

'Psychiatric drugs are no more capable of ridding me of my supposed delusions than they are of making atheists out of religious fanatics or communists out of free thinkers.'

Could this person be trusted to take the medicine prescribed for him?

The second account reveals the opposition of a patient diagnosed as schizophrenic, a term that encompasses a much larger area of mental disorders today than it did 50 years ago. She was given Stelazine.

'The drug put me almost in shock. Many thoughts flashed through my mind. My eyes were glazed. I was dizzy... After two weeks on that drug I flushed the rest of it away.

'Other addictive, mind-bending drugs were forced on me in three different psychiatric units...

'They come after you with a needle. You hit the nurse, you knock the needle from her hand. She gets another dosage. They bring in more orderlies...'

As a former psychiatric nurse, I can relate to this account. The mentally ill today are no different than the ones I dealt with. The medications have changed and they do provide relief for many more than we were ever able to help.

The problems caused by the return to the community of the medicated persons must be faced and overcome. We must financially support community health centers in providing emergency services, out-patient and in-patient care, and consultation services. We must recognize the need for more board and care homes, halfway houses, communal housing and single room accommodations.

The alternatives are that the unwanted may end up at a flophouse, on the streets or in jail. The question may be, what would caring relatives choose, the alternatives, or hospitalization? Will society improve in its attitude toward the mentally disturbed? Will we see more neighborliness, more humanitarianism, more tolerance?

In the 1930's one of our nurses tried an experiment in giving a patient a normal environment, with nearly fatal results. Carmack, the Scottish nurse I had worked with on H4, was fulfilling a lifelong ambition to move to a farm, renting one in the Fraser Valley. With consent of the Administration at Essondale, she arranged to take Albert, a parole patient, as a farm helper. She would pay him pocket money and give him freedom from institutional life.

Carmack's rented farm was not far from the one where I grew up, and where my parents were now living again. They hadn't been able to find anyone willing to rent, and they could not keep two places going any longer. At least they could produce food for the table though there was still little money to be made in farming.

Gladwin had come out with me for a couple of days off, and we visited Carmack, who was relaxed and happy in a large, gracious home. "My two nephews are here on week-ends," she said. "They'll be able to spend the summer and help with the haying. Albert manages the cows and gets the milk to the station." The B.C. Electric interurban line went right by her place so she could ship milk, potatoes and other produce into town. "As long as I can pay the rent, I'm happy with this life," she said.

We found Albert working around the barn, and he showed us the room fixed up for him in one of the sheds. "Everything I want," he said, beaming.

Gladwin and I went to a dance that night in the community hall, and there was Albert, smiling and good-looking with his rosy cheeks and dark, curly hair, making a big hit with the girls. He came over immediately and danced with each of us in turn, then went back to the girls who were falling over one another trying to impress the new young fellow they knew only as the farm helper for Miss Carmack.

"Shall we tell them?" I mused. "Evidently Carmack hasn't told the neighbors where he's from. I'd feel kind of guilty spilling the beans." We decided not to say anything. Albert was having such a good time, and after all, that was the idea, wasn't it?

"He does seem stable," Gladwin said. "But those girls will have to learn that you can't go by looks. You have to know a man's background."

I was no longer at the hospital when I saw Carmack again after a harrowing experience with Albert.

"I should have known!" she said. I had heard the story from my parents as it was known far and wide, but I was hearing Carmack's own reactions. "I'd taken him back to Essondale a couple of times before, when he was starting to act queerly, but this time I left it too long. I was just getting too used to him, I guess."

Carmack was alone in the house one Saturday night. Her nephews had gone to a movie. She went to bed before they came home, but when she heard the back door open she knew by the unnatural silence and the stealthiness of the footsteps that it was not Alex and Bruce. Albert was not to come in the house except for meals.

"I knew it was him," she told me, her face quivering with the memory of her fear, "and I knew he'd gone over the edge. I was out of my bed and out the window without even putting on slippers, and I ran up the road in my nightie and bare feet to the neighbor's to phone the police. I must have pounded on that door for five minutes before they answered and let me in. I was so afraid the boys would come home and walk into the house before the police got there, and be faced with a madman."

Police found her room in a state of disorder that only a lunatic frenzy could produce.

"He'd piled clothes from my closet and from my dresser drawers on top of the bed," Carmack told me. "Then he dumped my chamberpot all over everything. They found him upstairs hiding in a closet in the boys' room. He had taken a pair of scissors apart and had slashed the boys' pillows into shreds. He'd slashed my pillows too." She shuddered. "He meant to kill us. I get nightmares yet."

"Did the police have any trouble with him?" I asked.

"No, strangely enough he handed over the scissor blades and they took him away, and that's the last I've seen of him. You can be sure I never took him back and I won't try anyone else from there either."

Unexplained violence that takes the life of individuals or of whole families, hatred that results in assault and rape---evidences of emotional instability are before us daily. Yet properly understood, ideally by the person so afflicted, an onset of deep depression can be endured and a period of euphoria used to great advantage. The life of Dr. Clare Hincks serves as an example, early in this century.

Dr. Hincks knew he was manic-depressive. Before the antipsychotic medications which would have made his suffering less severe were known, he 'descended into a living hell' at regular intervals. He also rose to heights of euphoria with high spirits and bursts of energy not typical of the average person, yet he did good work as a doctor in the field of psychiatry, improving conditions for those who were confined in mental hospitals in the early part of the twentieth century.

As the General Director of the National Committee for Mental Hygiene, Dr. Hinks set up training centers for psychiatrists and psychiatric nurses in Brandon, Manitoba, which became a model across the continent. Through his teachings, caring and therapeutic methods were gradually introduced into mental hospitals. Preventive services were set up in communities and psychiatric clinics established.

Dr. Hincks became General Director of the National Committee for Mental Hygiene in Canada and eventually held that position for the United States. All this because Dr. Hincks recognized his own condition and used his periods of superhuman brilliance and energy to achieve more than the ordinary person could do.

In 1948 Dr. Ryan, as Medical Superintendent of Essondale, made a tour of mental hospitals across Canada and in the United States, and met with Dr. Hincks. His report reads:

"Spent about three hours with Dr. Hincks gaining considerable enlightenment and insight into the sphere of mental hygiene. He expressed much pleasure and interest in activities at Essondale and congratulated the administration and staff on its apparent success."

Certainly improvements had been made from the days in the not too distant past when insane asylums confined the unfortunately afflicted in dark, unsanitary cells and brutal treatment was all too common. Yet many questions remain to be answered today. How useful is psychoanalysis? How dangerous are the drugs in use? Are the dosages correct, and how often are they not taken by unsupervised individuals? Should some of the dangerous characters at loose be hospitalized, who are not? When someone with a history of violence is jailed, is the sentence too short? Should parole be given? Has the pendulum swung too far in the direction of freedom?

And what is to be done about the street people, who sleep in doorways or under bridges?

Obviously the perfect solution to the problems of mental illness has not been reached as yet. The institution which protected society from the vagaries of the unsound mind, and protected these people from themselves, has been replaced by chemical compounds and community facilities which are hard-pressed to handle the load. Much remains to be done.

In looking back at my three years as a psychiatric nurse, so many years ago, I marvel at the carefree attitude which we maintained in an essentially dangerous occupation. And I realize that the key I carried was the key to a view of human behavior such as few people ever get to see or imagine.

* * * * * * * * *